# English in Medical Education

## LANGUAGES FOR INTERCULTURAL COMMUNICATION AND EDUCATION
**Series Editors:** Michael Byram, *University of Durham, UK* and Alison Phipps, *University of Glasgow, UK*

The overall aim of this series is to publish books which will ultimately inform learning and teaching, but whose primary focus is on the analysis of intercultural relationships, whether in textual form or in people's experiences. There will also be books which deal directly with pedagogy, with the relationship between language learning and cultural learning, between processes inside the classroom and beyond. They will all have in common a concern with the relationship between language and culture and the development of intercultural communicative competence.

Full details of all the books in this series and of all our other publications can be found on http://www.multilingual-matters.com, or by writing to Multilingual Matters, St Nicholas House, 31-34 High Street, Bristol BS1 2AW, UK.

# English in Medical Education

An Intercultural Approach to Teaching
Language and Values

**Peih-ying Lu and John Corbett**

**MULTILINGUAL MATTERS**
Bristol • Buffalo • Toronto

**Library of Congress Cataloging in Publication Data**
English in Medical Education: An Intercultural Approach to Teaching Language and
Values/Peih-ying Lu and John Corbett.
Languages for Intercultural Communication in Education: 24
Includes bibliographical references and index.
1. English language—Medical English—Conversation and phrase books (for medical
personnel). 2. Medical personnel—Language—Conversation and phrase books (for
medical personnel). 3. Medical personnel and patient—Language—Conversation and
phrase books (for medical personnel). 4. Transcultural medical care—Language—
Conversation and phrase books (for medical personnel). 5. Communication in medicine. 6. Medicine—Language. I. Lu, Peih-ying. II. Corbett, John, 1959-
PE1127.M4E44 2012
428.0071–dc23 2012021843

**British Library Cataloguing in Publication Data**
A catalogue entry for this book is available from the British Library.

ISBN-13: 978-1-84769-776-9 (hbk)
ISBN-13: 978-1-84769-775-2 (pbk)

**Multilingual Matters**
UK: St Nicholas House, 31–34 High Street, Bristol BS1 2AW, UK.
USA: UTP, 2250 Military Road, Tonawanda, NY 14150, USA.
Canada: UTP, 5201 Dufferin Street, North York, Ontario M3H 5T8, Canada.

The policy of Multilingual Matters/Channel View Publications is to use papers that are
natural, renewable and recyclable products, made from wood grown in sustainable for-
ests. In the manufacturing process of our books, and to further support our policy, prefer-
ence is given to printers that have FSC and PEFC Chain of Custody certification. The FSC
and/or PEFC logos will appear on those books where full certification has been granted
to the printer concerned.

Typeset by Techset Composition Ltd., Salisbury, UK.

# Contents

# Acknowledgements

We wish to express our gratitude to various institutions and individuals who supported us in the writing of this book. The Royal Society of Edinburgh and the Taiwanese National Council of Science generously made a travel exchange award available in 2010 for Lu to travel from Kaohsiung to Glasgow to discuss the early stages of the project. In the later stages, a Start-Up Research Grant from the University of Macau enabled Corbett to visit Taiwan. We would like to thank the students at Kaohsiung Medical University who gave us inspiration and opportunities to think about possible ways of delivering language courses, and colleagues at KMU and at Glasgow University in the College of Arts and the College of Medical, Veterinary and Life Sciences, for their enthusiasm and contribution of ideas in the writing process; in particular, Dr Wendy Anderson, Christine Borland, Dr Catherine Emmott, Professor Christian Kay, Professor Chung-sheng Lai, Carole Macdiarmid, Professor Alison Phipps, Alna Robb and Dr Jer-jia Tsai. The authors are also grateful to Professor John Skelton who read a draft of the complete manuscript and, alongside encouraging comments, pointed out numerous gaps and infelicities and suggested many improvements. The staff at Multilingual Matters were unfailingly helpful and patient. Special thanks also go to Augusta Alves, who patiently supported us throughout the long gestation of this volume. The responsibility for any faults that remain lies, of course, with ourselves.

The authors and publishers acknowledge the following sources of copyrighted materials and are grateful for the permissions granted. While every effort has been made, it has not always been possible to identify the sources of all the materials used, or to trace all copyright holders. If any omissions are brought to our notice, we will be happy to include the appropriate acknowledgements in future editions. *Un Leçon Clinique à la Saltpêtrière* (1887) by André Brouillet is reproduced by kind permission of the Musée d'Histoire de la Médecine, the Université Paris Descartes; *The Anatomy Lesson of Dr. Nicolaes Tulp* (1632) by Rembrandt van Rijn is reproduced by kind permission of The Royal Picture Gallery, Mauritshuis, The Hague; and *A Loving Skin-graft*, by Shi-Qiao Li is reproduced by kind permission of Kaohsiung Medical University. Permission to reproduce screenshots of the TIME corpus was kindly given by Professor Mark Davies of Brigham Young University.

# 1 Introduction – English in Medical Education

This book explores the many interactions between recent and current developments in medical and language education. It will be of most relevance to those who are involved in teaching English to medical students, but it should also interest those who are teaching English to practising healthcare professionals and those involved in developing cross-cultural competence in medical education. Some parts of the book may also be of use in designing courses in medical communication for native speaking medical students; it will be clear that we have drawn inspiration from descriptions of a number of such courses ourselves. There are, of course, many textbooks that are written to be used either in the teaching English for medical purposes (EMP) or in training proficient or native speaker students to communicate effectively in medical settings. However, these textbooks differ from each other in many respects and the present volume also offers a change of focus and direction from most of the books currently available. This introductory chapter surveys the current scope of EMP, explains why we believe a change of direction may be merited, at least in some educational contexts, and previews the contents of the book as a whole.

English, of course, has long been recognised as a basic requirement for medical training internationally (e.g. Maher, 1986), and medical schools in countries ranging from Poland to Singapore now advertise programmes in medical education that are fully or partly taught in English. Institutions in other countries include English language training as a component of a medical degree; in some Taiwanese medical schools, for example, language classes may form part of a General Education component that is taught for two years before a further five years of pre-clinical and clinical training begins. In other schools, EMP might be taught in parallel with the medical curriculum. Of course, in Anglophone countries, the intake of medical students now generally includes a substantial cohort of non-native speakers (e.g. Hayes & Farnill, 1993). Beyond the bounds of medical schools, too, large-scale migration of both health-care providers and their potential patients means that practising clinicians and their colleagues regularly face situations where English is being used as a lingua franca in consultations.

The teaching of English for medical purposes has arisen in response to these educational and professional pressures. The textbooks and learning materials currently available to teach EMP focus on different aspects of the discipline. Some target the language and skills that medical students require in order to read medical texts in English or to cope with the demands of a course taught partly or entirely in English. Others address the occupational demands of working in an Anglophone environment on practising physicians whose first language is not English.

The learning materials used in EMP courses are naturally shaped by the pedagogical assumptions that underlie them. To take a few typical examples, *The Language of Medicine in English* (Bloom, 1982) and *English for the Medical Professions* (Beitler & Macdonald, 1982) focus largely on reading skills as a means of acquiring medical vocabulary. There are nods towards other means of reinforcing the vocabulary thus encountered, by memorisation through structural drills and further practice via conversational interaction, but reading remains the core activity. Bloom (1982) is designed around 10 relatively broad topics, from 'Medicine, its History and Folklore' to 'Medical Emergencies' and 'Prevention and High Technology Health Care'. The structure of each unit is similar (Bloom, 1982: i):

Each lesson begins with a glossary of special terms in which specific vocational words and expressions are defined. There follows a vocabulary practice section in which questions and answers guide the reader to proper use of these terms. Then the terms are used again within a contextual frame of reference. Each section is followed by topics for discussion which give the student an opportunity to use special terms, structural patterns, and general vocabulary. The lesson ends with comprehensive vocabulary review and conversational practice.

Beitler and Macdonald (1982: i) also have reading as their primary concern, although their topics are more technical, including 'Genetics,' 'Anatomy and Physiology' and 'Chemistry,' and their stated aim is:

to bring students rapidly to a point where they can read medical texts of increasing difficulty and density with relative ease and a high degree of comprehension. Each reading is preceded by a rigorous vocabulary

presentation and drill, and followed by extensive reading and comprehension exercises.

Both textbooks are designed for learners who have already acquired a relatively high level of general English proficiency and who are now embarking
on medical studies.

By contrast, *Professional English in Use: Medicine* (Glendinning & Howard,
2007), *English in Medicine: A Course in Communication Skills* (Glendinning &
Holmström, 2005) and *Cambridge English for Nursing* (Allum & McGarr, 2010)
are all principally directed at learners who are already practising professionals, though they may also be of use to students in the pre-clinical and clinical
phases of their training, especially when the students are interacting with
patients. Glendinning and Howard (2007) shares with the other textbooks
described above a primary concern with teaching medical vocabulary.
Designed mainly for self-study, it introduces practitioners to the terminology
associated with topics such as 'X-Ray and Computed Tomography (CT)',
'Epidemiology', and 'Screening and immunization'. However, part of this
textbook, like Glendinning and Holmström (2005) and Allum and McGarr
(2010), also deals with typical encounters in which listening and speaking
skills are more prominent. In medical settings, oral communication skills
include the ability to 'take a history', 'examine a patient', 'discuss a diagnosis', 'welcome a patient on admission', 'describe wounds' and 'show empathy'. The reading and writing illustrated by these textbooks also relate to the
overall goal of being relevant to working professionals: they include case
notes and forms, as well as medical journal articles. In many respects these
textbooks are similar to guides to medical communication that are aimed at
native speaker medical students, such as the popular textbook *Communication
Skills for Medicine*. The preface to this volume states its purpose thus (Lloyd
& Bor, 2009: i):

Many doctors increasingly recognise that communication skills in medical practice are not simply about positive engagement with patients.
Effective communication also helps us to understand better a patient's
problem, the impact it has on a patient's life and relationships and how
best to manage the problem in the patient's life. Nowadays, effective
communication skills are also vital for reducing the risk of error in clinical practice as well as avoiding complaints about one's practice. Both of
these could have serious consequences for the doctor.

Lloyd and Bor also organise their teaching units around communicative events
such as medical interviews and exchanging information; however, compared

to Glendinning and Holmström's textbook, Lloyd and Bor's volume brings to the fore those communicative situations that native speakers would find as difficult to handle as non-native speakers. These situations include breaking bad news, taking a sexual history, dealing with complaints, calming challenging patients, coping with personal issues and communicating with children and young people. Particularly relevant to the present volume's concerns is one chapter on 'Communicating with patients from different cultural backrounds', an issue also dealt with by two training DVDs designed for doctors working in a multicultural city (Moss & Roberts, 2003; Roberts *et al.*, 2008). The training DVDs attempt to raise practitioners' cultural competence by training them in conversational analysis and reflection. The use of language theory, in this case pragmatics and speech act theory, as a framework for reflection is also key to Skelton's (2008) discussion of language and clinical communication. Skelton's provocative contribution casts a sceptical eye over a 'checklist' approach to teaching communication skills, arguing that a whole-person approach to education is no less necessary than a whole-person approach to medicine.

Clearly, all of the types of EMP learning materials described have their uses. Medical students need to grasp the technical language of the discipline quickly; they need to be able to function effectively in the kinds of communicative situation that recur frequently in medical interaction; and they particularly need advanced communication skills to deal with difficult and stressful situations, where the emotional stakes are high. Their instructors need to embed the teaching of communication skills in the rich context of the students' own lives. We certainly do not wish to understate the continuing value of existing materials and courses; however, we feel that – except occasionally in passing – most of the EMP materials and courses of the kind illustrated by these examples manifest a curious absence. The passing references to 'empathy' and 'different cultural backgrounds' point to a potential direction for EMP that, particularly in medical education in a second language, has been relatively neglected (see, however, Candlin & Candlin, 2003).

In medical education, the direction to which we refer is usually called 'cultural' or 'cross-cultural competence' (e.g. Betancourt, 2003, 2004). In language education, its correlate is 'intercultural communicative competence' (e.g. Byram, 1997; Corbett, 2003; Risager, 2007). In these approaches to medical and language education, attitudes, values and beliefs are moved from the margins of pedagogy to occupy a much more central position. This position is sometimes expressed as 'professionalism' in medicine. Hafferty (2006: 2151) argues that the 'next wave' of professionalism demands qualities beyond clinical knowledge and 'outward behavior':

Being a physician – taking on the identity of a true medical professional – also involves a number of value orientations, including a general commitment not only to learning and excellence of skills but also to medical behavior and practices that are authentically caring.

It is our argument in the present volume that issues of 'cross-cultural competence' and 'professionalism' coincide with questions of attitude, value and identity in intercultural language education. As noted above, many medical students in today's world combine their clinical education with either pre-clinical general education or supplementary language classes, usually in English. Therefore, the purpose of the present volume is to explore the rationale for addressing intercultural communicative competence in medical education, and to suggest some ways in which the concerns of medical education might be practically addressed in the intercultural language classroom.

The correspondence between cross-cultural medical education and intercultural language education forms the substance of the second chapter in this volume. In this chapter, we take up the challenge set out at the outset of Candlin and Candlin (2003: 134):

> Applied linguists, and in particular those concerned with the analysis of discourse in professional contexts, would do well in our view to look outside their own professional literature for studies that direct themselves at health care communication, especially where this involves issues of intercultural communication.

As they go on to demonstrate, the professional literature in healthcare is rich in studies of intercultural communication, and they note the 'discursive turn' taken by sociologists of medicine (ibid: 142). What interests us most in Chapter 2, however, are the resonances between cross-cultural competences and intercultural communicative competence as curricular goals in medical and language education respectively.

A brief survey of literature on discourse and intercultural communication can be found in Corbett (2011). This overview notes the distinction sometimes made between studies of communication that are 'cross-cultural' and those that are 'intercultural'. The former compares communication in one culture with that in another; for example, patterns of communication in a television programme that exists in different international formats might form the basis for a cross-cultural comparison of versions across cultures (cf. the discussion of Western and Asian patterns of discourse in the quiz show, *The Weakest Link*, in Cheng and Warren, 2006). Intercultural communication, on the other hand, is arguably concerned with what happens when people from a given culture interact with people from other cultures. While this terminological distinction may be useful, it is not generally observed in the medical literature, where 'cross-cultural communication' generally refers to interactions between people from different cultural backgrounds, as is evident from the following excerpt from a medical article on cross-cultural competence (Betancourt, 2003: 546):

Sociocultural differences between patient and physician influence communications and clinical decision making. Evidence suggests that provider-patient communication is directly linked to patient satisfaction and adherence and subsequently to health outcomes. Thus, when sociocultural differences between patient and provider aren't appreciated, explored, understood, or communicated in the medical encounter, patient dissatisfaction, poor adherence, and poorer health outcomes result. It is not only the patient's culture that matters; the provider's "culture" is equally important.

In the present volume, then, 'cross-cultural' and 'intercultural' communication are regarded as largely synonymous, as they are in much of the medical literature. When 'cross-cultural' is used in the present volume, it simply suggests that the source of the issue being discussed is in the medical rather than the applied linguistics literature.

Studies of intercultural communication are themselves diverse; they range from research into communicative styles and values associated with broad cultural groups (e.g. Trompenaars & Hampden-Turner, 1998; Hofstede, 2005) to smaller scale empirical studies of particular episodes involving intercultural exchanges (e.g. Bailey, 2000). While we draw on many examples of intercultural interactions from the professional literature, our overall approach to intercultural language education is influenced by the work of pedagogical theorists and practitioners such as Michael Byram (1997, 2008) and Karen Risager (2007). This pedagogical orientation moves language education beyond a narrow focus on linguistic competence, and even beyond a concern with communicative skills and strategies, towards a wider conception of language ability that draws upon a knowledge and appreciation of different value systems (cf. Corbett, 2011: 314–315). Intercultural speakers can draw upon extensive understanding of different styles of interaction and cultural behaviour, they are politically aware, and they exhibit attitudes of openness and curiosity.

Byram and his colleagues have been influential in shaping that part of the *Common European Framework of Reference for Languages: Learning, Teaching,*

*Assessment* (CEFR) which deals with intercultural communicative competence. While the components of intercultural communicative competence are set out in some detail in Chapter 2, it is worth quoting here the CEFR's general statement about intercultural language education (Council of Europe, 2001: 1):

> In an intercultural approach, it is a central objective of language learning to promote the favourable development of the learner's whole personality and sense of identity in response to the enriching experience of otherness in language and culture.

At first glance, this statement may seem to have little relationship to the instrumental demands of cross-cultural training in medical education, as outlined by the quotation from Betancourt, above. However, it seems to us reasonable to suggest, at least, that there is a demand for healthcare professionals who are disposed to regarding encounters with 'otherness' as 'enriching', and whose sense of personal and professional identity has been shaped by positive engagement with people from other cultures. In other words, we believe that the attitudes, values and beliefs that form the core of intercultural communicative competence are cognate with those that are articulated in the medical literature as 'cross-cultural' competence – and it is this relationship that we explore more expansively in Chapter 2. Effectively, we argue that the literature on cross-cultural competence in medicine enhances and deepens our understanding of intercultural communicative competence in healthcare settings. Together, they provide a curricular basis for our intercultural approach to teaching English in medical education.

If Chapter 2, then, defines the 'what' of our approach, Chapter 3 addresses the 'how'. After the so-called 'methodology wars' of the last century, English language teaching has moved into what has sometimes been characterised as a 'post-methods' phase (e.g. Kumaravadivelu, 1993, 2006). The label is, perhaps, unfortunate, since even 'post-method' forms of language education assume that there are more and less effective ways of teaching and learning a language. However, current language pedagogy seeks to resolve potentially unhelpful conflicts between teaching for communicative fluency and teaching for structural accuracy by focusing instead on classroom tasks that learners are required to perform (Kumaravadivelu, 2006: 65; original emphasis):

> It is precisely because a task can be treated through multiple methodological means, Kumaravadivelu (1993) argues, that TBLT [task-based language

teaching] is not linked to any one particular method. He reckons that it is beneficial to look at task for what it is: a curricular content rather than a methodological construct. In other words, different methods can be employed to carry out language learning tasks that seek different learning outcomes. Using a three-part classification of language teaching methods, he points out that there can very well be language-centered tasks, learner-centered tasks, and learning-centered tasks. *Language-centered* tasks are those that draw the learner's attention primarily to linguistic forms. Tasks presented in Fotos and Ellis (1991) and in Fotos (1993), which they appropriately call grammar tasks, come under this category. *Learner-centered* tasks are those that direct the learner's attention to formal as well as functional properties. Tasks for the communicative classroom suggested by Nunan (1989) illustrate this type. *Learning-centered* tasks are those that engage the learner mainly in the negotiation, interpretation, and expression of meaning, without any explicit focus on form. Problem-solving tasks suggested by Prabhu (1987) are learning centered.

Corbett (2003) asserts that TBLT is an appropriate means of developing intercultural communicative competence, the extra-linguistic goals of which can be incorporated seamlessly into learning-centred tasks. However, it is the reference to Prabhu (1987) which may resonate with those involved in medical education. In the late 1960s, McMaster University Faculty of Health Sciences developed a new medical curriculum based on 'problem-based learning' (PBL) thus initiating a wave of curriculum reforms in medical schools around the globe (Barrows, 1996). Though its global growth in popularity has resulted in different variations being practised, PBL in medicine generally engages its students in experiential group learning tasks (for an overview, see Albanese, 2010). One PBL cycle, over several class meetings, might require students to address a fictional case study, brainstorm possible ways of researching it, pursue those lines of research, present their findings, refine their research, present further findings and then suggest possible treatments (see further, Chapter 3). Where medical education is delivered through the medium of English, students may be required to engage in this activity in their second language. PBL cycles can also be seen as complex problem-solving tasks in Prabhu's (1987) understanding of the expression, that is, PBL involves a series of language activities (e.g. brainstorming, prioritising, researching and presenting, evaluating and recommending) that are directed towards a non-linguistic goal (i.e. recommending a treatment for a particular ailment). Chapter 3, then, explores the fruitful resonances between TBLT and PBL as a potential way of achieving the goals of an intercultural curriculum in medical education.

It may, however, with justification, be argued that any language curriculum should pay attention to the enhancement of language awareness, and the enrichment of the learner's linguistic resources. In intercultural language education, the continuing concern with a narrow conception of 'language' is sometimes called 'languastructure' (Risager, 2007). Chapters 4 and 5 take two complementary approaches to the teaching of medical languastructure. Research into medical language has, in the main, either focused on written academic texts in medicine (e.g. Nwogu, 1997), or it has centred on the discursive practices that characterise doctor–patient interactions (for a brief overview, see Halkowski, 2011). Chapter 4 addresses concerns in the teaching of medical language, while Chapter 5 samples some of the extensive literature on 'medical talk', and suggests some implications for teaching.

A problem for teachers of medicine is in deciding what kind of language is representative of the medical domain; for example, Hyland (2002) argues persuasively for a high degree of specificity in teaching any academic discipline, which means that students of dentistry, anatomy and nursing should be exposed to and master different sets of texts from those in other branches of medicine. While we are deeply sympathetic to genre-specific teaching, we recognise that we cannot cover the full range of medical genres here – nor can any individual course in medical English. We argue that a useful compromise, particularly in the earlier stages of medical education, is to raise students' language awareness of technical terminology while contrasting the specialised vocabulary of 'medical' registers with everyday expressions about disease and associated medical concerns. In Chapter 4, therefore, we consider language-centred tasks (cf. Kumaravadivelu, quoted above) that encourage students actively to exploit online resources (both of medical and general language), and reflect on the use of the terms in academic and non-academic domains. This kind of activity we see as preliminary to more focused, genre-specific language tasks based on the students' own particular sub-disciplines.

Chapter 5 turns to the issue of medical talk. Shi (2009: 212) comments that:

> Compared with research on written medical genres, which focuses on the structure of discourse based on analyses of lexical items, semantics, syntax, and rhetorical organization, studies of spoken genres focus on the impact of social, political and cultural dimensions of medical communication on language use. By focusing on communication as social practice, EMP applied linguists have examined how oral interactions differ and unfold based on the strategic use of language by people marked with status differences, such as doctors, nurses and patients.

Indeed, Li goes on to dub this focus of research activity 'English for sociocultural purposes', and the concerns raised by this branch of applied linguistics lie close to the heart of the present volume. Chapter 5 is indeed the most extensive of the chapters in this book; even so, it can only sample much of the rich research in the medical and applied linguistics literature in its consideration of intercultural exchanges between the different kinds of interlocutor (doctors, nurses, patients, family, friends, caregivers, translators) who, in different configurations, may be involved in face-to-face medical communication.

The subtitle of this book is 'An intercultural approach to teaching language and values', and, as we observed above, the distinctive feature of intercultural language education, as we see it, is its willingness to address the impact on communication of different cultural systems of value, attitude and belief. While values are embedded in medical discourse, a prerogative of intercultural language education is that space should be made in the curriculum to reflect upon them, as well as on the other values that constitute the medical student's developing professional identity. Chapter 6 therefore considers the issue of 'critical cultural awareness' in the context of medical education. Here, we draw upon the sociology of medicine and critical medical anthropology to devise ways of interrogating the mainstream values that characterise professional biomedicine. Respect for different value systems and sympathy for different beliefs about medicine, both professional and non-professional, are intercultural resources that assist clinicians in the negotiation of appropriate treatments with patients from diverse backgrounds.

Chapters 7 and 8 continue the themes of language and values in medical education by drawing inspiration from the realm of medical humanities. The past decades have seen a considerable growth in the medical humanities as universities, particularly in the USA and UK, strive to dissolve perceived barriers between subject areas, and medical educators seek ways of addressing human values in biomedical practices (Gordon & Evans, 2010). There is a longstanding debate about whether medical practice is essentially a science or an art; in truth, it is both. Clinicians obviously draw upon scientific knowledge when treating illness, but also must craft a personal relationship with patients and colleagues in order to practise effectively. The distinction is expressed in Chapter 6 in terms of 'curing' a disease by the application of clinical expertise, and 'healing' the patient by attending to the significance and impact of the illness in the wider context of their lives. In medicine, the expertise that is necessary to 'heal' as well as to 'cure' usually comes from years of accumulated experience that may not yet be available to young medical students, who are often from relatively privileged backgrounds. The arts are one means of gaining access to a culture's pool of experience intensely and dramatically, if at a vicarious remove.

In language education, of course, literature has long had an established, if sometimes contested, place as a means of engaging learners to enhance their linguistic repertoire. Chapter 7, then, reviews the case for the use of literary texts in both language and medical education, and illustrates some ways of using them with medical students, both to improve language skills and address the human issues that healthcare professionals need to be able to consider. Charon (2000) goes so far as to argue that the skills used in literary analysis are transferable to the professional domain; effective clinicians draw upon what Risager (2007: 229) calls the 'poetics' of the language as a resource with which to understand the nuances, inferences and lacunae evident in medical communication.

Chapter 8 extends this discussion into the realm of the visual imagination. As with literature, the visual domain has long been recognised as a valuable resource in language education (e.g. Goldstein, 2009). Some courses in medical humanities (e.g. Boisaubin & Winkler, 2000) use fine arts, both as a point of access and stimulus to encourage observational skills and to encourage discussion of the human issues that are often on vivid display. In some cases, artists have been invited to work with medical students to discuss overlapping interests in medicine, communication and the arts (cf. Lu, 2010). The chapter ends with a consideration of the pedagogical use of television and film dramatisations of medical subjects; combining both literary and visual qualities, these art-forms are popularly used in medical education, though some practitioners raise questions about their value (e.g. Czarny et al., 2010). As Chapters 7 and 8 attest, we see literature and the visual arts as invaluable resources in intercultural language education (cf. Byram & Fleming, 1998), combining opportunities for meaningful language engagement and spaces for critical reflection on medical issues.

Finally, Chapter 9 reviews issues of course design in relation to intercultural language education in medical contexts. We are aware that the present volume is far from a recipe book for ready-made courses in English for Medicine. Rather, it seeks to articulate a rationale for an intercultural approach to teaching English in medical education, alongside some practical possibilities for classroom teaching. Everyone's course will differ, and rightly so. Nevertheless, Chapter 9 offers guidance in course design, by rehearsing the basic considerations that must be addressed in relation to the intercultural approach we advocate: considering the environmental constraints, articulating the perceived students' needs, identifying curricular goals, sequencing content, presenting the materials, monitoring and assessing student achievement, and evaluating the course. We illustrate these considerations in relation to illustrated examples drawn from our own experience. We do not pretend to have designed a series of successful EMP courses that can stand as shining paragons for the benefit of others. Indeed, the present volume is born of our frequent frustration at having designed or observed courses that fall short of our aspirations. On these occasions we console ourselves with the words of Samuel Beckett (1983: 7): 'Ever try. Ever fail. Try again. Fail again. Fail better'. Indeed, as we suggest in Chapter 9, one of the most important components in course design is often one of the most neglected: the analysis of environmental constraints (Tessmer, 1990). To illustrate this point, and conclude this introduction, we offer the follow-ing vignette, a condensed version of different episodes that we have observed. We had been invited by an institution to act as consultants in the evaluation and future development of an EMP course. As part of this process, we talked to staff and students, and observed a sample lecture:

We are in a large lecture theatre in an Asian university. The room's capac-ity is 130 and there are about 100 students present. It's 10 am. The sub-ject of the lecture is Medical Vocabulary. The students are in the second year of a 7-year degree programme; their attendance at this course is compulsory. At the front of the lecture theatre is a doctor in a white lab coat. He conducts the lecture largely in Chinese with the aid of power-point slides, a laser-pointer, and a microphone. He has an engaging, jovial style of delivery. The content of the lecture is the vocabulary of different anatomical systems: he indicates points on the slides and translates the technical terms for the chest (thorax): 'sternum', 'clavicle', 'rib', etc. He gives no further context for the terms, at least in English. The students sit in rows, elevated towards the back of the lecture theatre. They have workbooks in front of them; some have laptops. The lecturer demon-strates pronunciation (the –tion endings of 'respiration', 'ventilation' etc) and he occasionally interacts with the students: he calls on individual students from a list; not all the students on the list are present. The interactive activities vary slightly; e.g. the lecturer asks students for an alternative name for the clavicle: 'collarbone'; he does word-building drills (pleura – pleuritis, and so on).

Some students leave and enter as the hour drags on. Those who remain seated are involved in different activities. Some are reading a list of medi-cal terms that they have downloaded from a medical website,[1] others are studying a cloze-like activity in their workbook: 'A cardiologist is a doctor for the _____ .' Some are taking notes in pencil; some are reading and annotating printed versions of the power-point slides. The less studious are checking their email accounts; some are drawing cartoons; some are talking to other classmates; a few are fast asleep.

Not surprisingly, this course was the topic of some debate within the institution: it had recently been introduced, and it had been the butt of complaints from both students and the medical lecturers who were assigned to deliver it. To us as observers, it was unclear what the purpose of the lectures was: each hour introduced a multitude of new terms. Were the students seriously expected to memorise them, and assimilate their meaning and pronunciation within the space of 60 minutes? Was the lecture intended to guide home study?

In discussion with the members of staff who had to deliver the courses, it was clear that they shared our confusion about the aims of the course, but it also became clear that many of the problems with the course stemmed not from any rationale for course design, but from environmental constraints. For various administrative and logistical reasons within the institution, this course had been assigned to medical lecturers, who presented the sessions in rotation, though English language teachers were employed by the institution for other courses. Indeed, the English language teaching unit was supposed to advise the medical lecturers on content and modes of delivery. However, the medical lecturers did not give the language course a high priority in their teaching, and so did not devote enough time to master the materials that the language unit provided. While cross-disciplinary team-teaching is often advocated in English for Specific Purposes, it can be difficult to manage in practice. Meanwhile, our discussions with the students suggested that they sat dutifully through most of the sessions, sometimes taking it in turns to attend and take notes, and that they used a combination of power-point print-outs and web-sourced materials to swot up on the targeted vocabulary shortly before the multiple-choice examination.

In this kind of situation, any English teacher, course designer or consultant may not be able to produce a glib 'intercultural' solution from a hat. It is relatively easy to gain colleagues' agreement on the shortcomings of courses; it is not always easy to find and implement an agreed solution. In the illustrative case, time had to be spent rebuilding trust across the cultural divide between medical teaching staff and the language teaching unit. We as consultants could only add our voices to the debate between the university administrators, medical teaching staff and language unit, and point to possible alternative ways of delivering appropriate language courses. To a great extent, the present volume has emerged from our thinking about just such alternatives.

## Note

(1) On inquiry, we later learnt that the website was 'The Merck Manuals' a medical site now available at http://www.merckmanuals.com/home/index.html [Retrieved 5th October 2011]

# 2 Intercultural Communicative Competence in Medical Settings

This chapter reviews the sometimes contested but still useful notion of 'competence' as a concept that guides curriculum development, with specific reference here to intercultural language education and medical education. We survey some of the major competence-based models of the 'intercultural speaker' and the 'cross-cultural medical practitioner' in these two pedagogical domains, with a view to identifying areas of common concern as well as difference. Finally, we allude briefly to some of the challenges to competence-based models of education that have been raised by critics such as Barnett (1994) and Phipps and Levine (2010), in anticipation of a fuller discussion in later chapters. In brief, in this chapter we give an overview of:

- Models of intercultural communicative competence in language education, developed by educationalists such as Byram (1997, 2008) and Risager (2007), and now embodied in policy documents such as the *Common European Framework of Reference for Languages: Learning, Teaching and Assessment* (Council of Europe, 2001). This multinational, plurilingual set of guidelines has as its North American counterpart the American Council for the Teaching of Foreign Languages' (1996) *National Standards for Foreign Language Education: Preparing for the 21st Century*. Both sets of curricular guidelines seek to address the acquisition of intercultural as well as communicative competences.
- Models of cross-cultural competence in medical education, such as the American Association of Medical Colleges' (2006) *Tool for Assessing Cultural Competence Training* (TACCT). As its name suggests, the TACCT resource is designed as a means to identify whether medical education

courses are facilitating the development of knowledge and skills in cross-cultural communication.

There are reservations about the rise of 'competence' as an educational goal; Barnett (1994) critiques its relevance to tertiary-level education in general (see Chapter 6) while Watson *et al.* (2002) question the reliability and coherence of 'competence-based' models of nursing education. Despite these reservations, one of the general aims of tertiary education is still regularly expressed as a means of equipping students with the knowledge and skills necessary to address cultural diversity. Often this aim is expressed in terms of understanding and respecting difference. For instance, Harvard University's (2007) *Report of the Task Force on General Education* recommended that its students should develop their cultural awareness, for example by studying a non-Western culture. The task group's rationale is expressed as follows (Harvard University, 2007: 16–7):

The influence around the world of the United States culturally, economically, militarily, and scientifically is unprecedented. Yet, for that very reason, it is difficult for students inside the United States to understand this country from an international perspective, as a nation in continuous engagement with societies around the world, sometimes cooperatively and sometimes confrontationally. Students may be easily persuaded, by the manner in which other societies are represented in the press and in the culture of public life, that other people are, in some universal sense, "essentially" Americans. An important aim of the courses in the Societies of the World category is to help students overcome this parochialism by acquainting them with values, customs, and institutions that differ from their own, and by helping them to understand how different beliefs, behaviors, and ways of organizing society come into being.

In a similar vein, the president of Harvard at the time of the task force's report suggested in a critique of 'underachieving colleges' that today's students generally need to develop competences for 'living with diversity' and 'living in a global society' (Bok, 2006: 194–224, 225–254).

The move to address cultural difference in both language and medical education, then, can be contextualised in a set of more widespread concerns about 'parochialism', 'insularity' and the resultant misunderstandings that lead to conflict. The language learner is in a privileged position to cross borders and engage with cultural difference directly, while the medical student's engagement with cultural differences is envisaged as having ethical and practical benefits, such as greater equality of provision across ethnic, racial, class or gender divides, and increased patient 'compliance' with medical advice.[1] Consequently, practitioners in language and medical education have developed frameworks of intercultural and cross-cultural competence that characterise the knowledge, attitudes and skills that learners may draw upon. In the following sections, we review major models and draw comparisons between them.

---

### Task: Encountering otherness

Take a few moments to recall your own experience of teaching or learning a foreign language. Did the language classes directly address the different cultural behaviour of the speakers of the other language(s)? If so, how was this done?

- By explanation of the other culture, for example, by 'cultural capsules' of information?
- By readings in textbooks or illustration through film and television?
- By direct encounters with members of that culture, for example, teaching assistants, online correspondents, and so on?

How would you now describe the attitudes that you, or your learners, formed towards speakers of the other language(s)? Were they positive or negative, stereotypically predictable or surprisingly complex?

---

# Defining Intercultural Communicative Competence

The notion of 'competence' in language education has been subject to considerable refinement and re-evaluation for over half a century. The term was popularised in linguistic study by Noam Chomsky's dichotomy between 'performance' (what actual language speakers did) and 'competence' (what ideal language speakers *knew* in order to be able to do what they did; see, e.g. Chomsky, 1965). Chomsky's concern was principally with modelling an internalised grammar that would account for an ideal speaker's ability to produce grammatically correct sentences. While educationalists today are less focused on idealised standards of 'correctness', it is still fair to say that most language teachers aim towards increasing their learners' ability to use the target language in accordance with rules of accuracy, whether these be internationally exported or locally produced. Chomsky's 'linguistic competence' was quickly critiqued by the sociolinguist, Dell Hymes (1971) who coined the influential term 'communicative competence' to cover that which the language speaker has to know in order to use grammatically correct forms appropriately in situated contexts. Effectively, Hymes extended Chomsky's model to include rules of cultural behaviour as well as grammatical rules, and a further influential account by Canale and Swain (1980) included grammatical competence, sociolinguistic competence and strategic competence as component parts of an overall model of communicative competence. The language speaker has to know how to form acceptable utterances, and use them appropriately to accomplish their goals.

The focus of communicative competence, however, was on the norms and behaviour expected by and of native speakers of the target language. In the 1990s, as intercultural language education was devised and developed by Michael Byram and fellow educators such as Gerhard Neuner, Lynne Parmenter, Karen Risager and Geneviève Zarate (e.g. Byram *et al.*, 1997), the model of intercultural communicative competence sought to articulate the kinds of knowledge and skill required of speakers moving within and among *different* language communities, where linguistic norms and cultural values – and therefore social behaviour – are likely to vary. Moreover, if English is being learned and used as a *lingua franca* by people of different cultural backgrounds, what knowledge and skills should effective communicators be expected to learn, in order to negotiate these varying cultural attitudes and behaviours, and to mediate when conflicts and other difficulties arise? The Council of Europe's *Common European Framework of Reference for Languages* (hereafter CEFR) also seeks explicitly to address these issues from the outset, in a passage quoted earlier (Council of Europe, 2001: 1)

> In an intercultural approach, it is a central objective of language learning to promote the favourable development of the learner's whole personality and sense of identity in response to the enriching experience of otherness in language and culture.

This statement pushes the language learning agenda far beyond issues of grammatical correctness, contextual appropriateness or even the strategic accomplishment of social goals through language. Intercultural language education engages the learners' 'whole personality' by seeking to promote an 'enriching' encounter with 'otherness'. Models of intercultural communicative competence attempt to articulate those personal qualities that teaching should encourage, so that the learners' exposure to otherness can indeed be an enriching rather than diminishing experience.

---

## Task: Expressing goals

As a language teacher, reflect for a moment on what you normally expect your learners to be able to do at the end of a course. Write your goals as a list. Then classify them into groups:

- How many are expressed as features of grammar, vocabulary, pronunciation, discourse, and so on (i.e. language goals)?
- How many are expressed as skills (e.g. able to read, write, listen to or say certain things)?
- How many are content goals (e.g. able to demonstrate knowledge of particular topics)?
- How many are task-oriented (e.g. able to achieve particular goals)?

Would you consider any items on your list *cultural* goals? If so, how are they expressed?

This activity gives an insight into your presuppositions about what a language teacher in your educational context should be teaching. It is useful to note that there are various ways of envisioning a language teacher's role.

---

# Components of Intercultural Communicative Competence: *Savoirs* and Resources

In a major work on the specification of intercultural communicative competence, Byram (1997) developed a framework of what he called *savoirs*. Byram's proposed model consists of five separate but interdependent components: attitudes, knowledge, skills of interpreting and relating, and skills of discovery and interaction, which together lead to critical cultural awareness. Critical cultural awareness empowers students to voice their own opinions and facilitates the kind of personal growth that prepares them to be global citizens (see further, Byram, 2008). Most immediately, Byram's model can be used, as in the *Common European Framework of Reference for Languages*, to assist in the design of language curricula, the preparation of classroom materials and the conduct of classroom activities and learner assessment (see further, below). In this vein, Corbett (2003) explores the application and adaptation of Byram's model to English language teaching, and Corbett (2010) suggests some practical activities that address intercultural learning in the ELT classroom.

Despite subsequent criticism of their limitations, Byram's *savoirs*, then, remain a key point of reference for anyone considering the constitution of intercultural communicative competence. In brief, the five *savoirs* are listed below (for more detail, see Byram, 1997, 2008; Corbett, 2003; Neuner & Byram, 2003):

(1) *Savoir être*: Attitudes, curiosity and openness, readiness to suspend disbelief about other cultures and belief about one's own.
(2) *Savoirs*: Knowledge of social groups and their products and practices in one's own and one's interlocutor's country and the general processes of societal and individual interaction.
(3) *Savoir comprendre:* Skills of interpreting and relating: the ability to interpret a document or event from another culture, to explain it and relate it to documents or events from one's own.
(4) *Savoir apprendre/faire*: Skills of discovery and interaction: the ability to acquire new knowledge of a culture and cultural practices and the ability to operate knowledge, attitudes and skills under the constraints of real-time communications and interactions.
(5) *Savoir s'engager*: an ability to evaluate critically on the basis of explicit criteria, perspectives, practices, and products in one's own and other cultures and countries.

In Byram's formulation, the *savoirs* rework earlier models of linguistic and communicative competence, and add to them a positive attitude about encounters with linguistic and cultural otherness, a basic knowledge about different cultural values and behaviours, a set of ethnographic skills of discovery and interaction, and a critical stance about the production of knowledge and its dissemination by the education system. As noted, Byram's model has come in for extensive comment and some criticism. For example, Duffy (2002) and Belz (2003: 71) raise issues about the formulation of some of the *savoirs* as 'attitudes' and 'skills', noting that the extent to which specific classroom activities can be held responsible for the inculcation of qualities such as 'openness' and 'curiosity' remains under-researched. Rather, the causal connection between classroom activities and desired outcomes remains an article of faith for many intercultural language educators.

The nature of the *savoirs* has also been challenged and subjected to reformulation, for example by Karen Risager (2007) who suggests that they are less a set of characteristics of intercultural speakers and more an instrument of assessment, especially given Byram's involvement in embedding the *savoirs* into the CEFR. Risager (2007: 168–187) reshapes Byram's five-part inventory, offering a set of what she prefers to call 'resources' that theoretical intercultural speakers should be able to draw upon in interaction. Furthermore, she adds two more 'resources', those of 'linguistic identity' and 'poetics'.

Risager's reformulation of 'knowledge and skills' as 'resources' and her expansion of the components of intercultural communicative competence have their attractions. First, it is helpful to reconceive knowledge and skills as a potential set of resources that learners can draw upon with increasing confidence and sophistication. Second, the 'identity dimension' recalls aspects of Hymes' formulation of communicative competence in its concern with how a speaker might draw on aspects of sociolinguistic variation to project an identity that is recognisable with reference to the interlocutors' background knowledge and attitudes. And finally, the 'poetic' dimension focuses on the speaker's use of the literary qualities of language – oral and textual – to develop characteristic styles and narrative strategies. Through the 'poetic' dimension, the learner can take creative and imaginative owner-ship of the language being learned.

Risager's adaptation of Byram's model suggests not only its possible shortcomings, but also, more positively, its flexibility. Intercultural com-municative competence can be conceived as a dynamic set of qualities, which might usefully be supplemented and revised. The formulations that are offered as guidance to curriculum designers, textbook writers, teachers and assessors are just that – guidance – and should not be considered abso-lute categories for every educational context. Later in this volume, we shall consider the adaptation of intercultural communicative competence in the context of medical education. Before we turn to that, we consider in more detail two powerful, but still provisional, statements about linguistic and cultural competence, namely that of the CEFR, already referred to, and its American counterpart, the *National Standards for Foreign Language Learning: Preparing for the 21st Century* (American Council for the Teaching of Foreign Languages, 1996; see also National Standards in Foreign Language Education Project, 1999, 2006).

## Task: Teaching attitudes and values

Pause for a while and reflect on the implications of the foregoing section for your own language teaching practice. In particular:

- Have you previously considered the formation of *attitudes*, alongside skills and knowledge, to be part of your role as a language teacher?
- Do you think the teaching of attitudes and the values on which they are founded is actually part of the language teacher's role?

- Is the teaching of attitudes and values more likely to be part of the language teacher's role in a state school than in a commercial school?
- If they are to be taught at all, how should attitudes and values be integrated into language teaching? Should the teacher simply attempt to impose their worldview on learners?
- Who should determine the attitudes and values that are to be taught?

# Intercultural Communicative Competence: National and International Standards

The number of teachers who engage directly with models of intercultural communicative competence, as discussed in journal articles or books, is obviously limited. These discussions enter the broader educational discourse indirectly through national and international statements of good practice, such as the *Standards for Foreign Language Education: Preparing for the 21st Century* (American Council for the Teaching of Foreign Languages, 1996 and its successors; hereafter 'American Standards') and the European CEFR (Council of Europe, 2001). Though relatively few practising language teachers might read these lengthy and detailed documents, their influence on the profession is diffused via curriculum planning, undergraduate and postgraduate courses in education and applied linguistics, the design of textbooks, and discussions and demonstration at professional conferences such as TESOL and IATEFL. It is therefore worth considering their guidance as representative of current thinking on the relationship between the teaching of language and 'culture.' As major curricular guidelines, sponsored by established institutions, their impact is also evident beyond North America and Europe.

## The American Standards: Preparing for multicultural citizenship

The American Standards are explicitly designed to encourage teachers and learners to address the practices and engage with the products of diverse cultures as a way of 'decentring' from familiar perspectives and estranging familiar values. Cross-cultural engagement is embedded into language learning through a process of comparison and making connections between communities. Thus, the American Standards recognise that modern languages can be learnt through content-based courses on a variety of subjects, such as history, social studies, science and the fine arts. This approach helps students to 'develop an interdisciplinary perspective at the same time they are gaining intercultural understandings' (ACTFL, 1996: 12). Knowledge of a second language and culture combined with the study of other disciplines shifts the focus from language acquisition to broader learning experiences for the student. Overall, the American Standards emphasise both the linguistic and cultural insights that come with foreign language study and consider them as prerequisites for both living in a multicultural nation and in a globe imagined as a culturally diverse neighbourhood.

The teaching approach of the American Standards document is based on the '5 Cs', namely, communication, cultures, connections, comparisons, and communities (ACTFL, 1996: Appendix 3). Language learning is thus embedded in the broader concept of cultural learning. The guidelines state that 'the true content of the foreign language course is not the grammar and the vocabulary, but the cultures expressed through that language' (ACTFL, 1996: 43). Although communication is still considered to be at the heart of second language study, three major elements of the American Standards focus specifically on cultural learning: cultures, connections and comparisons. Learners will specifically engage with the following topic areas (ACTFL, 1996: 43–8):

• *Perspectives*: attitudes, values and ideas.
• *Practices*: of social interaction, and patterns of behaviour accepted by a society.
• *Products*: books, foods, laws, music, and so on.

In many practical ways the authors of the American Standards document accord, consciously or not, with the views of intercultural communicative competence that were developing throughout the late 1980s and 1990s. Indeed, Met and Byram (1999) categorise the cultural content recommended by the American Standards into familiar domains:

• Aspects of culture that can be learned factually.
• Knowledge about one's own culture.
• The acquisition of methods of cultural investigations and analysis.

Thus, the American Standards blends knowledge (of one's own and other cultural values, behaviour and products) with skills (of discovery, interpretation) in ways that echo the *savoirs* in attractively realisable ways. For example, the American Standards suggest that learners should be able to identify, discuss, and analyse tangible or intangible cultural products and be able to evaluate themes, ideas, and perspectives related to the product being studied (ACTFL, 1996: 12). Learners are also expected to explore the relationships among the products, practices, and perspectives of the cultures being studied.

The American Standards also stress the importance of learners knowing that people do not necessarily share the same culture just because they speak the same language; cultural boundaries do not necessarily coincide with linguistic isoglosses or national borders. In this respect, the American Standards recognise that cultural teaching should not simply provide a fixed image or set of reductive stereotypes of otherness; instead, teaching-and-learning language-and-culture is a process.

## A common framework for a plurilingual union

In Europe, a plurality of national and sub-national languages constitutes an essential feature of European cultural heritage; safeguarding this heritage and increasing access to it as a valuable shared resource are among the aims of the Council of Europe (Council of Europe, 2001: 2). As with the American Standards, the general aim of the CEFR is for learners to be able to deal with linguistic and cultural diversity. However, unlike its American counterpart, the Council of Europe is a trans-national body, concerned with harmonising distinct national identities within a larger imagined community. By acquiring some of the languages of other European member states, learners are expected to be able to exchange information and ideas with speakers of other languages, as well as to achieve a wider and deeper understanding of the perspectives and practices of fellow Europeans from different national traditions. The CEFR also explicitly indicates that among its pedagogical goals is the following aim (Council of Europe, 2001: 4):

> To promote methods of modern language teaching which will strengthen independence of thought, judgment and action, combined with social skills and responsibility.

In the CEFR, socio-cultural knowledge is broken into several specific concepts which are defined as distinctive features of a society such as everyday living, living conditions, interpersonal relations, value, body language, social conventions, and ritual behaviours, each with a set of descriptors (Council of Europe, 2001: 101–103). For example, everyday living includes food and drink, meal times and public holidays. Values, beliefs and attitudes cover issues such as social class, occupational groups, and regional cultures. The model of inter-cultural communicative competence explicitly owes much to Byram's *savoirs*. Emphasis is again placed on a combination of knowledge and skills generally, which here include specific formulations of competences such as know-how (*savoir-faire*) and 'existential' competences such as *savoir être* and *savoir apprendre*. Given less prominence in both the American Standards and the CEFR is

Byram's *savoir s'engager*, or critical cultural awareness, a topic that we explore in more detail in Chapter 6. Like the American Standards, the CEFR proceeds by promoting comparison and contrast; it suggests that learners should become familiar with 'life in the target community and essential differences between practices, values, and beliefs in that community and the learner's own society' (Council of Europe, 2001: 158).

Although they are expressed in rather different ways, the American Standards and CEFR guidelines share an assumption that language learning in the early 21st century is driven by a social imperative, namely to promote understanding of, and respect for, linguistic and cultural diversity, both within multicultural nations and across plurilingual borders. Their response to this imperative is to articulate intercultural communicative competence as the kinds of knowledge and skills that today's learners should ideally achieve to function in communities characterised by diverse languages, values and behaviours. In the apparently unrelated domain of medical training, a similar imperative, namely to promote understanding of, and respect for, the linguistic and cultural diversity among patients likely to be seen by trainee and practising physicians, has also promoted curricular reform informed by models of cross-cultural competence. Of course the two domains are not separate: as individuals experience greater physical mobility in contemporary society, as tourists, immigrants, refugees or temporary overseas workers or students, increasing numbers are likely to require medical attention at some point in their lives. Encounters between medical professionals and patients, all from diverse backgrounds, simply represent specialised cases of intercultural communication more generally, but ones in which the personal and emotional stakes can be extremely high.

---

## Task: National and international frameworks

Here, reflect for a moment, as a language teacher, on your own previous familiarity with the CEFR or the American Standards. Each is easily available online, in the latter case in summary form. Who do you think is their primary readership?

Have you found them *directly* useful or irrelevant to your practice as a language teacher? In particular, have you found their guidelines on integrating language and cultural knowledge to be helpful?

If you have had little or no direct engagement with these international frameworks, are you aware of their *indirect* impact on your practice, for example, through textbooks that you use, or language assessments that you prepare your learners for?

> Is the influence of the CEFR and American Standards limited to the USA and Europe alone? If you are not an American or European language teacher, are you familiar with other national or international frameworks that attempt to guide your practice?

## Models of Cross-Cultural Competence in Medical Education

Much of the literature on cross-cultural competence in medical education is specifically directed to addressing two discrete but related issues: (i) the disparities in medical provision between members of different cultural communities, and (ii) the promotion of shared decision-making about treatment. Betancourt (2003: 560) links these two issues:

> A growing literature delineates the impacts of sociocultural factors, race, and ethnicity on health and clinical care. Clinicians aren't shielded from diversity, as patients present varied perspectives, values, beliefs, and behaviors regarding health and well-being. These include variations in patient recognition of symptoms, thresholds for seeking care, ability to communicate symptoms to a provider who understands their meaning, ability to understand the prescribed management strategy, expectations of care (including preferences for or against diagnostic and therapeutic procedures), and adherence to preventive measures and medications.

Clinicians who are not prepared for cultural diversity may fail to take into account the impact of divergent beliefs, values and behaviour when patients present. As a result, misunderstandings may occur which result either in the clinician delivering inadequate levels of care or in the patient refusing or being unable to comply with the medical procedures negotiated or prescribed. An educational solution is to provide programmes that encourage medical students to develop into 'intercultural speakers' by promoting the acquisition of relevant competences. A widely used definition of cross-cultural communicative competence in medical education is based on Cross *et al.* (1989) and used by the Association of American Medical Colleges (e.g. AAMC, 2005: 1):

> Cultural and linguistic competence is a set of congruent behaviors, knowledge, attitudes, and policies that come together in a system, organization,

or among professionals that enables effective work in cross-cultural situations. "Culture" refers to integrated patterns of human behavior that include the language, thoughts, actions, customs, beliefs, and institutions of racial, ethnic, social, or religious groups. "Competence" implies having the capacity to function effectively as an individual or an organization within the context of the cultural beliefs, practices, and needs presented by patients and their communities.

Intercultural clinicians are thus constructed as professionals in a complex community of practice whose sensitivity to racial, ethnic, social and religious diversity reduces disparities in healthcare provision and enhances shared decision-making about treatment; it becomes part of the goal of medical education to develop adept intercultural communicators. Furthermore, in an influential monograph, Cross et al. (1989: 19) extend the application of cross-cultural competence from the individual clinician to the entire healthcare system and its stakeholders, identifying five desirable characteristics:

The culturally competent system values diversity, has the capacity for cultural self-assessment, is conscious of the dynamics inherent when cultures interact, has institutionalised cultural knowledge, and has developed adaptations to diversity. Further, each of these five elements must function at every level of the system.

Cross et al.'s definition of cultural competence is designed to enable each part of the organisation and community to come together to work effectively in the context of cultural diversity. The need for understanding of culturally conditioned communication styles is accentuated by research that suggests that high incidences of failure amongst medics from ethnic communities was not on the grounds of prejudice, but on the grounds of candidates' non-adherence to privileged discursive strategies (e.g. Wass et al., 2003).

In parallel with language education there has been a growing awareness in medical institutions that professional education needs to respond to cultural diversity; and one response has been to articulate the competences that are considered desirable for the effective intercultural communicator. Thus, in the United States, accrediting bodies increasingly request medical schools to include cultural training in their programmes (Kripalani et al., 2009), and in the UK, Tomorrow's Doctors: Recommendations on Undergraduate Medical Education (General Medical Council, 1993, revised 2003, 2009) also stresses that medical students should develop competence in 'communicat[ing] clearly, sensitively and effectively with individuals and groups regardless of their age, social, cultural or ethnic backgrounds or their disabilities, including when English is not the patient's first language' (2009: 21).

It is clear, then, that pedagogical literature discussing the need to develop cultural competence in clinicians and medical students – and other healthcare professionals – is now extensive (for further examples, see Rees & Ruiz, 2003; Dogra & Wass, 2006; Americano & Bhugra, 2010). There has been considerable discussion about the values that medical students may lack and so need to acquire in their training; for example, Roberts *et al.* (2008) report that medical students in two British universities demonstrated discomfort with issues relating to ethnic and cultural diversity, while Campinha-Bacote (1999) argues that nursing students need to develop a 'cultural desire' to empathise with and care for people from different cultures. There is some debate in the literature relating to the definition of key terms; for instance Kumaş-Tan *et al.* (2007) observe that some measures of cultural competence often equate 'culture' with race and ethnicity (rather than, say, gender or social class) and much guidance for the development of cultural competence focuses simply on exposure to and knowledge of people from different races and ethnicities. However, a substantial amount of the medical literature on cultural competence shares with intercultural language education an emphasis on the articulation of a set of appropriate attitudes, skills and knowledge (e.g. Betancourt *et al.*, 2003; Kripalani *et al.*, 2006; Seeleman *et al.*, 2009). Attitudes, knowledge and skills are used to classify three domains that Betancourt *et al.* (2003) identify in competence training:

- The cultural sensitivity/awareness approach: Focusing on attitudes.
- The multicultural/categorical approach: Focusing on knowledge.
- The cross-cultural approach: Focusing on skills.

These domains inform an exhaustively detailed inventory and questionnaire for the assessment of cultural competence training in medical schools, the *Tool for Assessing Cultural Competence Training*, or TACCT (AAMC, 2005, 2006; Lie *et al.*, 2006). Users of the TACCT questionnaire are encouraged to match the content of pre-clinical and clinical courses against 'domains' that include:

- The definition of cultural competence and its key aspects.
- The impact of stereotyping on decision-making.
- Awareness of health disparities.
- Cross-cultural skills, such as working with an interpreter.

Each domain has a set of detailed descriptors for the curriculum to follow. For example, in the domain of knowledge, students will be able to 'describe common challenges in cross-cultural communication (e.g. trust, style)'. Students whose training has covered the attitudes, skills and knowledge identified by the TACCT inventory, then, may be expected, by the end of medical school, to have acquired a satisfactory level of cross-cultural competence.

---

### Task: Evaluating TACCT

The TACCT inventory is available online in summary form (see AAMC, 2006). If you teach a course in medical language or communication, look at the checklist and note which of the domains listed are covered by your own course. Are there any gaps?

If you teach English in non-medical contexts, look at the TACCT checklist and consider if any of the skills, knowledge and attitudes on the TACCT list are relevant or can be adapted to other professional domains.

---

## TACCT and the *Savoirs*

The TACCT inventory can, in many respects, be seen as an elaborate extension of Byram's *savoirs* and Risager's 'resources', or a version of the CEFR or American Standards that has been devised for American medical educators. Indeed, many of TACCT's descriptors of knowledge, attitudes and skills can be related to Byram's formulations of intercultural communicative competence. For example, Byram's *savoirs* require learners to obtain knowledge of social groups and their products and practices in their own country. This corresponds to TACCT's requirements that students should be trained to identify the definition of ethnic groups and to define race, ethnicity and culture, including the culture of medicine. More specifically, Byram's *savoir s'engager* articulates the competent language learners' ability to evaluate, critically on the basis of explicit criteria, perspectives, practices and products in his or her own and other cultures. One part of this ability is the capacity to recognise and critically evaluate the effects of negative stereotyping of others. In Domain 2 of the TACCT inventory, courses in cultural competence are expected to train medical students to 'understand the impact of stereotyping on medical decision-making.' The TACCT toolkit draws upon a wealth of medical literature that recognises the issues of negative stereotyping in healthcare; for example, Betancourt (2006: 989) cautions against broadly applying stereotypes to individuals who apparently fall into categories such as 'the Hispanic patient'. Teal and Street (2009: 536) also discuss specific strategies to counteract stereotyping, which they acknowledge as a natural human process. They recommend a focus not primarily on the cultural group to which a patient nominally 'belongs' but on 'core cultural issues':

> Core cultural issues which physicians should be taught to recognize and assess include beliefs about gender roles, physician authority, physical space, family roles, beliefs or practices about death, religious beliefs, and explanations of disease (Davidhizar, Giger, & Hannenpluf, 2006; Rapp, 2006). Communication is also a core cultural issue with several aspects, including recognition of status (e.g., use of first names), non-verbal behaviors (e.g., the meaning and use of gestures), and communication styles (e.g., what is considered rude or overly direct speech).

Another example of TACCT's competences that relates to *savoir s'engager* can be found in Domain 3, which suggests that competence training should encourage students to:

*   recognize physicians' own potential for biases;
*   recognize physician-patient power imbalance;
*   describe potential ways to address bias.

TACCT contains some descriptions of competences that are specific to the medical profession and cannot be related so easily to intercultural communicative competence, for instance, knowledge of the 'epidemiology of population health', or skills such as 'diagnosis, management, and patient-adherence skills leading to patient compliance.' Nevertheless, it is fruitful to compare models of intercultural communicative competence with inventories of cross-cultural competence used in medical education since they are mutually enriching. Byram's *savoirs* and Risager's 'resources' identify general areas of everyday intercultural communication that are supportive in negotiating and mediating between cultures; the TACTT inventory and others like it suggest how such general formulations of attitude, skill and knowledge might be adapted and extended to particular circumstances, such as medical communication.

However, even granting the utility of an extended and adapted list of intercultural knowledge, skills and attitudes, tailored to the specific needs of healthcare professionals, there is still a reductive element to the specification of cross-cultural or intercultural communicative competence as an inventory of knowledge, attitudes and skills. Approaches to intercultural language education that are driven by inventories of resources, *savoirs* or cross-cultural medical knowledge, skills and attitudes may be in danger of reducing complex, situated, learned expertise to a more or less nuanced set of abstractions. Furthermore, although inventories like TACCT and the CEFR are valuable in developing curricula and in assessing training programmes, because they are an attempt to formulate *what* medical students should learn, they have little directly to say about *how* the competences will be acquired by students (we turn to the issue of pedagogical tasks for the acquisition of intercultural communicative competence in medical training in Chapter 3). As noted at the start of this chapter, the very notion of competence-based education in tertiary education has been critiqued by educationalists such as Barnett (1994). Barnett argues that tertiary education is essentially a site where students can develop critical reflection, which may include the freedom to question the very values on which their education is based. We explore critical reflection, which is indeed addressed in Byram's *savoir s'engager*, in more detail in Chapter 6. Other educationalists, such as Phipps and Levine (2010: 11), follow Byrnes (2006) in preferring the notion of 'capacity' to 'competence'. They note Byrnes' anxiety about the label 'competence' prompting a now unhelpful dichotomy with 'performance' (cf. Chomsky 1965, referred to above), and they continue:

> [...] beyond the theoretical and terminological distancing from older debates, how is 'capacity' really different from competence? We suggest that it is the disposition for action, not just about how well someone can do something but with competences subsumed beneath it. It is the *capacity for creativity and collaboration*, which is above all what foreign language education should expect of learners.

While acknowledging that the articulation of desirable curricular goals as competences is pedagogically valuable, for example in the assessment of programmes, Phipps and Levine call for educators to remember that the language classroom is a space for dynamic action – a space where teachers and students can embark on voyages of discovery, voyages in which they will reconstruct themselves through encounters with otherness. The following chapters in the present volume seek to bear this rallying cry in mind.

The pedagogical literature on cultural competence in medical education is mostly written in Europe, Australia and the United States; however, the issues that gave rise to it are even more widely relevant, although local conditions and priorities will vary. Taiwan is one instance of an Asian country experiencing the cultural diversity that results from the immigration of foreign labourers and inter-racial marriages, and there is inevitably an impact on healthcare provision and medical education. Furthermore, medical education globally is increasingly delivered partly or wholly in the medium of English, and, as more healthcare practitioners take advantage of international mobility, and encounter patients from different cultures, the development of what we are calling intercultural communicative competence is an internationally recognised issue in medical training (e.g. Kachur & Altshuler, 2004). In the case of Japan, Taiwan and Korea, for example, medical schools typically offer undergraduate programmes lasting six or seven years. These often consist of General Education and Basic Science courses, followed by pre-clinical training and finally clinical training (referred to as clerkships or internships). Some medical schools offer a fast-track postgraduate programme that may omit all or part of the General Education component. A common challenge for medical schools is how to integrate the teaching of intercultural communicative competence in English with medical education throughout the curriculum. This chapter has sought to address this challenge by surveying the nature of intercultural communicative competence in medical settings, while acknowledging the limitations of a competence-based educational model. The following chapters will take our argument forward by:

- comparing current modes of teaching both language and medicine;
- exploring the medical humanities as a potential resource for teaching language and addressing the values identified by models of intercultural communicative competence.

## Note

(1) The expression 'patient compliance' is now often replaced by 'concordance', 'shared decision making' or 'adherence' ( Skelton, 2008: 21, 71). Henceforth, we generally use the latter term to indicate the negotiation of treatment between practitioner and patient.

# 3 Task Design in Language and Medical Education

In Chapter 2, we surveyed the curricular goals of intercultural language learning and sought parallels with the development of an agenda to teach cross-cultural competences in medical education. A statement of desirable curricular goals, such as the CEFR, the American Standards or TACCT, may imply possible ways of attaining them, but it does not necessarily determine teaching and learning practices. Consequently, in this chapter we move from a consideration of the curricular goals of intercultural language learning in the context of medical education, to some of the key principles in designing classroom tasks with a view to attaining the goals of intercultural communication in medical settings. We address the following topics:

- The rationale for task-based learning in intercultural language education.
- A comparison of task-based learning in language education and problem-based learning in medical education.
- The process of developing language learners into reflective practitioners.
- How to implement task-based learning in intercultural medical communication.
- Sample reflective tasks for medical communication in the intercultural language classroom.

## Task-based Learning in Intercultural Language Education

In his introduction to intercultural language education, Corbett (2003) suggests that teachers adapt the familiar principles of task-based language learning (TBL) to the goals of the intercultural curriculum. TBL has been widely described as a robust 'post-methods' means of delivering language education (e.g. Kumaravadivelu, 2006), a means that focuses less on dichotomies such as 'teaching for accuracy' versus 'teaching for fluency' in favour of forms of experiential learning that may address a variety of goals. TBL is concerned with designing classroom activities that may be directed towards achieving enhanced language awareness, a range of communicative goals, or indeed the components of intercultural communicative competence that are formulated by the *savoirs*. This chapter restates Corbett's position, while focusing on the specific context of developing intercultural communicative competence in medical education. In brief, we argue that the procedures of task-based language learning are well-matched to the goal of developing intercultural communicative competence in medical settings, and, moreover, TBL has a number of useful parallels with the prevailing use of problem-based learning (PBL) in medical education. In the present chapter, we review the principles of task-based learning, compare TBL and PBL, and discuss how they can be harnessed in classrooms where medical students are being taught language and communication skills.

The literature on TBL is now well-established, though, as several commentators note, the principles underlying TBL are so broad as to allow competing definitions of what exactly is involved in a communicative task (e.g. Willis & Willis, 2001; Van den Branden, 2006). Van Den Branden (2006: 6–9) helpfully tabulates previous definitions of language learning tasks, before offering a clarifying synthesis and description (emphases as original):

> Classroom tasks should facilitate meaningful interaction and offer the learner ample opportunity to process meaningful input and produce meaningful output in order to reach relevant and obtainable goals. In other words, tasks invite the learner to act primarily as a language *user*, and not as a language *learner*.

Thus put, the notion of a language task seems uncontroversial: teachers would normally expect to give learners opportunities in any language classroom to interact meaningfully to reach some kind of obtainable goal. However, the distinctive feature of TBL is that the design and accomplishment of communicative tasks becomes the central feature of language courses and the element around which curricula are developed. In many language classrooms, and in many language courses, there is still an assumption, whether tacit or explicit, that much of the time should be devoted to the explanation, demonstration and practice of linguistic *forms*, whether these are presented as grammatical structures (e.g. question forms, tense and aspect, modal auxiliaries) or as linguistic functions (e.g. requesting, relating a narrative, making suggestions). In TBL the focus is centrally on the communicative task, and the assumption, supported by empirical research into second-language classrooms, is that by accomplishing this task, learners will draw on, extend and improve their available linguistic resources. In practice, TBL demands a reorientation of classroom practice to focus on what is being done, rather than what language might be used to accomplish the task. In medical communication, the distinction might be seen in Table 3.1.

Taking an example from Table 3.1, a teacher might choose to present and practise conditional clauses alongside other means of expressing hypothetical situations (e.g. 'If your wife knew you had come here today, how would she react?'; 'If you were in your wife's position, what would you do?'; 'It would be helpful to think about what to say to her.'). Typically, a language teacher would contextualise such utterances, give some controlled practice, and then devise a role-play or other activity in which learners might use hypotheticals 'freely'. In a task-based approach, typically, the teacher might ask the learners to consider how a doctor might deal with issues arising from a patient wishing to keep treatment a secret (cf. Lloyd & Bor, 2009: 135–138). The learners might role-play a dialogue between a doctor and a man who wishes to keep his treatment secret from his wife, using whatever linguistic resources they can draw upon. The teacher then might review the learners' performance, drawing attention to ways of enhancing their linguistic performance. Lloyd and Bor (2009: 137) suggest that:

> Asking future-oriented and hypothetical questions is a non-confrontational device that that will help some patients to consider ideas that they might otherwise fear to address.

Having indicated ways of enhancing learners' linguistic repertoire, the teacher can encourage them to integrate newly presented and familiar language

**Table 3.1** Form-based versus task-based learning

| Focus on language form/function | Focus on task |
| --- | --- |
| Question forms; asking and answering questions | Interviewing a patient |
| Imperatives; giving commands | Prescribing a course of action |
| Future with 'going to'; expressing intention | Informing a patient of treatment he or she is about to receive |
| Past tense narrative; telling a story | Taking a history |
| Conditional clauses; hypothesising | Dealing with problems related to secrecy |

in a related task, such as role-playing a dialogue between a doctor and a younger patient who wishes to keep the recommended treatment secret from his or her parents. Role-plays are, of course, a routine element of most language courses, whether the focus of the course is general or special purpose communication (e.g. DiNapoli, 2003).

In this example, the difference between form-based and task-based instruction may perhaps seem superficial, a matter of ordering and nuance. However, the advocates of TBL argue that the process of *beginning* with the task and then inputting necessary language at a later stage helps promote acquisition more effectively, since the learners are continually *integrating* new language with familiar language in the context of purposeful activity, rather than being encouraged to 'add on' new bits of language to their repertoire, for reasons that may be withheld until late in the lesson.

Tasks, broadly conceived, then, are of various kinds, and indeed, as we hinted earlier, 'post-methods' educationalists now argue that an inclusive definition of a classroom task will include form-based investigations of the language, as a kind of 'consciousness-raising' or 'metacommunicative task' (e.g. Rutherford, 1987; Wills & Wills, 2001: 173–174). Classroom activities that directly focus on formal accuracy rather than fluency indeed have their place in the language learning curriculum, and we do suggest ways of exploring medical language directly elsewhere, particularly in Chapter 4. Nevertheless, we agree with Wills and Wills (2001) that TBL is most usefully discussed when the goals of communicative tasks are non-linguistic in nature. Task-types are various, and may include the giving and following of instructions or directions, or taking part in simulations and role plays. A more extensive list is discussed below. In order to accomplish tasks, learners ideally draw unpredictably and creatively on the linguistic resources at their disposal. Their language will no doubt depart from the norms and targets expected by the teacher; and so a certain amount of 'scaffolding' (Nunan, 2004: 35) will be required to supplement and enhance the learners' linguistic resources. The art of teaching, as Nunan observes, becomes a question of judging how much scaffolding is necessary, how to work it into the class, and when to remove it.

Some teachers may remain uncomfortable with TBL precisely because, at face value, its goals are non-linguistic. Indeed, if language acquisition is to occur in TBL, a cyclical procedure is necessary in which the learners will attempt to fulfil the task, and perhaps attain their goals provisionally or partially. There then has to be a reflective phase whereby the teacher and/or the learners' peers *do* input more sophisticated language that would help the learners attain their goals more fully. This linguistic input will no doubt need to be explained and practised in context. The task, or a variation of it, can then be repeated to allow learners the opportunity to integrate any new language into their accomplishment of the task. Courses then revolve around cycles of related tasks, later tasks building on the earlier ones by virtue of what is sometimes called 'task dependency' (Nunan, 2004: 35).

This brief sketch of TBL should be sufficient to suggest its attraction to intercultural language educators. The exploration of culture, ethnographically conceived in terms of Byram's *savoirs* or Risager's 'resources' can be integrated into a language learning programme, as a set of non-linguistic outcomes by which to direct its language-acquisition activities. The two sets of curricular goals – cultural exploration and language development – are not necessarily entwined, but they are complementary partners, and their union in a task-based language curriculum that is informed by intercultural goals should result in intercultural communicative competence. We address this issue in more detail below. First, however, we compare TBL in language learning with an increasingly popular means of delivering medical education, namely problem-based learning (PBL).

# TBL and PBL

In the previous chapter, we considered how the goals of the intercultural language curriculum mapped onto the partly analogous goals of cross-cultural competence in medical education. The latter can be conceived of as a specific articulation of the general goals of developing intercultural communicative competence in language education. A similar mapping of educational practices can be seen between TBL and a now common, if still controversial, way of delivering medical education, namely PBL. There are differences between the two approaches: TBL in part follows from a theoretical position that argues that language acquisition occurs 'naturally' in an environment in which learners are engaged in accomplishing meaningful tasks through language. Language educators generally assume that the process of acquisition is 'naturally' triggered by meaningful interaction towards a purposive end. PBL does not quite follow from a theoretical position that proposes that the acquisition of medical knowledge is naturally triggered by accomplishing meaningful medical tasks in classroom environments. However, there are some broad correspondences between PBL and TBL, most strikingly the assumption that students learn complex content and skills most effectively, not when they are subjected to information-rich lectures, supplemented by personal reading, but rather when, supported by a facilitator, they are engaged in problem-solving activities towards a particular end. In this respect, both PBL and TBL fall into the broad category of 'experiential learning' that Barnett (1994) sees as characteristic of higher education's recent increased responsiveness to education for work and the professions.

Pioneered at McMaster University in Canada in 1969, PBL has since taken diverse forms in regions beyond North America and Europe (e.g. Mpofu *et al.*, 1998; Khoo, 2003). However, there are various similarities across the board, as Lee and Kwan observe (1997: 153):

> In a typical PBL tutorial, students are presented with clinical information on a patient. Students go through the process of problem identification, hypothesis generation, the generation of learning issues, and setting of group and personal learning objectives. It is not important for the students to come up with the correct diagnosis or treatment, but to use the clinical problem as a focus to acquire the knowledge in order to meet the learning objectives [...].

To illustrate this general pattern in more detail, at Kaohsiung Medical University in Taiwan, where PBL is run alongside more traditional lectures, a PBL cycle usually lasts six hours, made up of three two-hour sessions (Chen *et al.*, 2008). In the first session, the tutor presents the group of about 10 with a case study that acts as a 'trigger'. A chairperson and record-keeper are selected from among the students: the chairperson directs the discussion, with some possible input from the tutor when necessary. The students then make hypotheses and identify learning issues. For example, in the first session, if they suspect diabetes, they might consider the regulation of glucose and insulin, and complications such as hypertension. They then go off and research those topics online or in the library, and, in the second session, they present and discuss their results in groups, after which they identify further learning issues. These are researched in turn, and, in the final session, the students present their overall findings, draw conclusions and suggest courses of action.

Such a PBL cycle, then, involves a complex series of language tasks: the chair has to nominate speakers and allocate duties orally; the record-keeper has to listen, take notes and summarise ongoing discussions; the students have to read the 'trigger' (i.e. the complaint and attendant data, e.g. history, test results, initial management, clinical course of treatment and suggested resource list), make hypotheses and statements, find and read relevant literature on the topic, and present this orally to the group, no doubt using slides, photographs, graphs and other visual data. They have also to make deductions and recommendations – all possibly in their second language, English, if that is the medium of instruction. The facilitator, in turn, has to listen to the developing discussions and intervene if they believe something crucial is being neglected – if only to say, 'Is there anything else you haven't thought of?'

Some of the more controversial issues of PBL echo those in TBL. For example, there is an anxiety among some medical educators that PBL-based courses are unstructured, do not guarantee coverage of necessary topics, and fail to show progression; educators worry that too much time is spent on talking in tutorials and that the learning lacks depth; some argue that students are learning problem-solving techniques, not medicine per se (Lee & Kwan, 1997: 154). As in TBL, issues of 'authenticity' also arise. In language class there is a perennial debate about whether 'classroom tasks' can or should emulate 'real world tasks' for which they serve as potential rehearsals. Long and Crookes (1992), for example, argue that TBL syllabuses should be formulated on the basis of language tasks that are directly related to real world tasks. In the literature on PBL, an analogous debate centres on whether the PBL 'triggers' are rich and complex enough to function as adequate rehearsals for 'real world' complaints. Consequently, there has been a move towards 'real patient' PBL triggers, based on actual case studies, rather than triggers designed specifically for tutorial use (e.g. Dammers et al., 2001; Diemers et al., 2007; Stjernquist & Crang-Svalenius, 2007). Advocates champion 'real patient' PBL on the grounds of the relatively complex and unpredictable nature of the problems posed, and the motivational value of having students address 'actual' cases. Pre-clinical encounters with authentic case studies, according to Dammers et al. (2001), help students to acquire transferable relevant knowledge and critical appraisal skills when facing new sets of events. In addition, 'real patient' PBL fosters in students the qualities of responsibility and empathy through active engagement with the problems encountered by actual patients.

To summarise so far, then, powerful movements in both language education and medical education put the 'task' at the centre of the teaching process. In language learning, TBL presupposes that language learners' engagement with meaningful activities, in which non-linguistic goals are achieved through the use of language, will stimulate cognitive processes that enhance acquisition. PBL supposes that the complex series of tasks involved in the PBL cycle, especially when based on actual case studies, increases student motivation and promotes the acquisition of knowledge, as well as problem-solving skills. The two educational methodologies – TBL and PBL – are clearly complementary: language educators in medical contexts where English-medium PBL is used can break down the PBL cycle into clearly defined language tasks that can (i) prepare learners for engagement in PBL tutorials and (ii) enhance their general language acquisition. However, neither methodology in itself is necessarily intercultural – though each has the potential to be. In the following sections, we consider how TBL and PBL can be adapted to address specifically intercultural issues.

## Intercultural Problem-based Learning

As we argued in the previous section, the typical PBL cycle can be broken into a series of language tasks that can be rehearsed in the language classroom. Nunan (2004: 41–73) offers a useful checklist and extensive discussion of the basic elements of communicative tasks that can be used in the design of learning materials: goals, input, procedures, teacher's role, learners' role and settings.

Goals are the teacher's statement of what he or she intends the student to learn from the task. Goals are not to be confused with learner outcomes (since what the learner actually learns will be unpredictable), but they offer a crucial rationale for the task. Nunan draws on Clark (1987) to suggest that goals might be communicative in nature (e.g. exchanging information or opinion), sociocultural (e.g. to do with the everyday life of the target speech community), about learning-how-to-learn (e.g. setting realistic learning objectives) or focused on language and cultural awareness (e.g. promoting understanding of the systematic structure and functions of the language in context). To this list we might add *intercultural* communicative objectives, based on the development of the *savoirs* or intercultural communicative resources discussed in Chapter 2 (cf. Byram, 1987; Corbett, 2003; Risager, 2007). A task in a medical language class might therefore have the goal of developing a sense of how doctor-patient interaction works in different cultures (for further discussion see Chapter 5), or exploring how a medical professional might 'decentre' to make communication with a child more effective and empathetic. In a PBL scenario, an intercultural task might have the goal of moving beyond a clinical understanding of a complaint, to a broader discussion of how the patient's values, attitudes or beliefs might affect the way they negotiate an agreed course of treatment. The last two examples are developed in further detail below.

Input 'refers to the spoken, written and visual data that learners work with in the course of completing a task' (Nunan, 2004: 47). In a PBL scenario, input may take the form of materials used as a 'trigger' for discussion, research and presentation, namely, the case history and attendant documentation. This kind of material can also be used in the medical language classroom. However, to go beyond the purely informational or clinical content of medical data, learners may also be encouraged to look at narratives and stories told by patients and fellow professionals (see further Chapter 4), as well as literature and the visual arts (see Chapters 7 and 8). Similarly, news stories and extracts from non-fictional material such as diaries and memoirs (e.g. Weston, 2009) might be used explicitly to address the values, beliefs and attitudes that constitute intercultural communicative competence. Ideally, as noted above, input should not be designed purely for the language classroom, but should draw on 'real world' or 'real patient' data, to promote a sense of 'real world' complexity and relevance to the learners' needs.

Procedures, or classroom 'activities' (cf. Nunan, 1989: 10–11), specify what learners are expected to do with the input inside or outside the classroom. Again the issue of 'authenticity' can be raised; classroom procedures may be designed as rehearsals for other activities, whether these are PBL cycles in medical education or encounters between medical professionals and their patients or peers. The kinds of procedures involved in language tasks have already been previewed in this chapter and are often discussed in the pedagogical literature (e.g. Richards & Rodgers, 2001); however, a general, but far from comprehensive, list bears repeating. The activity-types listed below overlap to some extent, and some tasks can be seen as constitutive of others:

- *Information-gap*: information is communicated from one or more learners to another individual or group.
- *Information-sharing*: learners may share different kinds of content related to a particular complaint.
- *Problem-solving*: learners respond to a problem by sharing information and suggesting a plan of action.
- *Decision-making*: learners are given a problem for which there are several possible solutions and they must choose one through discussion and negotiation.
- *Opinion exchange*: learners are invited to have an open-ended discussion and exchange of ideas, e.g. about a story, poem or work of visual art. They do not need to agree on an outcome.

The communicative tasks listed above are all relevant to intercultural language learning, so long as the goal of the task is directed towards developing some aspect of intercultural communicative competence, and the input and activities support this goal. Thus learners may share information about different cultural attitudes to illness, with a view to later using that information to inform a case study about a person from a particular cultural group. Or a decision-making task may address areas of cross-cultural competence; for example, what pain-killers might be prescribed to a white, middle-class American female in her 40s, in comparison with a black, working-class

American male in his late teens or an immigrant, Korean shopkeeper in his late 30s, if they all present with similar symptoms, and have a similar health insurance provision.

Teachers' and learners' roles address the parts that learners and teachers are expected to play in the language classroom. Much of the discussion about teachers and learners' roles revolves around the degree of responsibility teachers and learners take for the delivery of learning outcomes. A more 'teacher-centred' approach will involve teachers determining course content, in accordance with curriculum guidelines, and dominating classroom interaction, as 'ringmasters' (Nunan, 2004: 69). Many teachers draw much of their professional identity from demonstrating their mastery of content and consequently leave little space for the learner to take an active role in the educational process. Equally, many learners expect teachers to be able to demonstrate their mastery and they may not value input from peers or other sources. A more learner-centred approach might have learners negotiating course content and goals with the teacher, and the teacher guiding students towards their achievement of their desired outcomes (cf. de Jong, 1996). Learner-centred teaching is more of a collaborative partnership between learners and teacher, with the teacher devolving some of the responsibility for learning – and consequently some of his or her authority – to the learners. In recent years, language teaching theory has favoured a more 'learner-centred' approach, partly because research into the nature of the 'good' language learner has highlighted certain characteristics that they are supposed to share. 'Good' learners tend to be self-directed, to be organised and creative, to seek learning opportunities and to be able to live with uncertainty. They are likely to learn from their errors, use their knowledge of the linguistic system strategically, actively use context and their world-knowledge to construct meanings, make intelligent guesses, focus on fluency and vary their style of speech and writing as appropriate to the situation (Nunan, 2004: 65–6; Benson, 2002; Griffiths, 2008). Although most teachers would recognise this description of the 'good' language learner as a happy ideal, they would no doubt acknowledge that many learners have to be trained to take responsibility for learning, particularly if the learner is culturally disposed to expect teachers to act as authority figures.

Even if an idealised 'good learner' can be extrapolated from research, expectations about teachers' and learners' roles vary across cultures and, even within cultures, across educational institutions. Age and maturity also affect learning processes and strategies. The good primary or secondary school learner is obviously different from the good learner in higher education. In medical education, there is some debate about whether Asian students perform well in PBL scenarios because they are said to expect education to be teacher-led rather than student-led, and issues of deference and modesty might prevent individuals from contributing effectively in discussion. Hussain *et al.* (2007) report on PBL sessions in Asian universities where learners shared information effectively but avoided 'critical engagement', which, the authors suggest, was due to a cultural tendency to avoid challenging the tutor or one's peers. They suggest that 'a new type of academic socialisation' may be necessary if Asian students are to take full advantage of PBL tutorials, a claim that, if true, impacts on language learning (Hussain *et al.*, 2007: 770):

> If students are introduced to the idea that critical thinking is a foundational concept of PBL, and then taught, for example, the art of rhetoric and argumentation (see Gokhale, 1995; Anderson *et al.*, 2001), then, although this activity may be seen to lie outside established cultural practices, it would permit new critical skills to be brought into tutorial work and overcome the cultural norms that mitigate against this. Such a move would require students and tutors to value the idea that significant disagreement and challenge in academic debate can be acceptable and beneficial. Again, students would need empowering to do this, and to be given the space to develop appropriate skills and dispositions.

Given its focus on critical cultural awareness, the intercultural language classroom might well be the place to develop 'critical skills' that can be transferred to other learning contexts, such as PBL sessions (see further, Chapter 6). These skills will involve shifts in the roles played by teacher and learner, and their mutual responsibilities can become an explicit area for classroom discussion.

Settings refers to the 'classroom arrangements specified or implied in the task' (Nunan, 2004: 70). Nunan distinguishes between 'modes' and 'environment.' The former may range from individual work to whole-class activities, with different arrangements of pair or group-work in between. The latter refers to the actual teaching situation, whether in a typical classroom, with seating in serried ranks or in a horse-shoe arrangement, or in other spaces. Increasingly, educators are blending classroom-based learning with online education (e.g. O'Dowd, 2007), and project-based tasks explicitly aim to extend the learning process from the classroom to the wider community. PBL cycles take the seminar room as the focus for a set of individual and group-based activities that spill over to internet and library-based research between sessions, in preparation for clinical work in hospital, after the pre-clinical phase is over.

Goals, input, procedures/activities, teacher and learner roles, and settings are, then, the basic elements of TBL, and these may be adapted to serve the

needs of an intercultural language curriculum, in this case one that is specifically targeted towards the medical profession. As we have seen, the core
assumption is that by immersing learners in tasks that need to be accomplished using language, we can develop their linguistic skills, intercultural
skills and medical skills. We shall shortly consider some sample tasks that
illustrate tasks that address intercultural communicative competence in
medical contexts. First, however, we wish to turn to a general critique of a
skills-based model of competence, to determine whether we can integrate
lessons from that more sceptical appraisal into our task design.

In his discussion of the relationship between higher education, knowledge and society, Barnett (1994) questions the move towards experiential
learning and the prevalent discourse of 'skills' and 'competence', at least at
university level. His argument is that an exclusive focus on skills and competence represents the undue influence of professional and workplace priorities on the traditional domain of higher education, which privileges critical
thinking within and across disciplinary specialisms. Barnett (1994: 63)
observes, by way of illustration:

> The practice of medicine and the academic discourse called 'medicine'
> may be about disease and the treatment of patients, but the two dis-
> courses are different. The practical discourse is about wrestling prag-
> matically with all the medical, interpersonal and ethical issues presented
> by individual patients to busy practitioners lacking most of the desirable
> resources; the academic discourse is about forming truth claims, hypo-
> theses and theories, and presenting evidence for critical scrutiny by
> one's peers.

Barnett himself goes on to question the sharpness of this distinction: one
traditional role of higher education is to prepare professionals for medicine,
the law and the church, for example, and 'the interpersonal and ethical
issues' faced by medical professionals may also be informed by 'truth claims,
hypotheses and theories', as well as the presentation of evidence for critical
scrutiny by one's peers. But Barnett's fundamental point is that, at its highest level, education should be about more than merely the acquisition of a set
of skills that may comprise an idealised 'competence', whether that is conceived of as medical, cross-cultural or even intercultural communicative competence. Barnett argues for space in the higher education curriculum for
'critique', 'understanding' and 'wisdom', which are all qualities that, he
argues, militate against the pre-ordained determination of a set of normative
standards and behaviours that function as a statement of competence. The
teacher's role, in Barnett's view, is as a 'subversive' (Barnett, 1994: 108):

[The teacher's] main purpose is to lessen the hold that any one form of understanding has on the student. [. . .] The student then comes to realize that there are always counter-claims that can be brought against any one position, but is still able to transcend that stage and go on take up a reasoned position of her own. The educator's task is to promote an understanding that is held, perhaps with some passion, but against a deeper understanding that this *is* a particular position that might have to be yielded sometime; as Goodlad (1976) put it, to develop a state of 'authoritative uncertainty.'

Only by developing a view of understanding as 'authoritative uncertainty' can a space be made for the generation of new knowledge, and new understandings that might indeed overtake those of the educator or curriculum designer. Barnett's recommendation for implementing this subversive role for teacher and learner is through allying critical reflection to the concept of 'experiential learning' that informs methodologies like TBL and PBL. Barnett (1994: 109) is sceptical about the phrase 'experiential learning':

[. . .] since *all* learning has to derive from some kind of experience; it is either stating the obvious or trying to demarcate certain kinds of experience as especially worthwhile. Even so, the idea of experiential learning does contain the important truth that we learn things and come to know things without always being aware that we have learnt or that we know. That is why much time is spent, where experiential learning is prized, in getting individuals to reflect on their experience so as to identify and bring into full consciousness what they have learnt.

It might be argued that, over the last two decades, formulations of learning goals, procedures and the competencies they seek to develop take Barnett's recommendations into account. For example, Nunan (2004: 37–38) advocates 'reflection' as a key stage in TBL, arguing that learners who understand the rationale for their learning will be more effective learners. Corbett (2003: 61, 67) includes an 'opportunity for reflection' as an important element in task design, not just to make learners conscious of their learning, but to give them a space to evaluate it; for instance, to consider whether the kind of conversational behaviour they have been practising is the kind of cultural behaviour they would be comfortable adopting. Furthermore, Byram (1997, 2008) and others have stressed 'critical cultural awareness' – which involves reflection and evaluation – as one of the principle components of intercultural communicative competence. Even so, Barnett reminds educators that higher-level learning cannot and should not be reduced solely to a set of curriculum statements and formulaic methodological procedures, useful though these undoubtedly are as provisional guides to educational practice. The gaining of understanding, as opposed to skill, is a hard-won achievement, involving many hours of reflection on a rich set of experiences, in which the rigid positions of the learners, their peers, and the tutor may all be challenged and tested through rational discussion. In practical terms, the intercultural teacher should be open to challenge and seek opportunities for discussion that will, on many occasions, confront his or her own deeply held values.

The foregoing sections have described the elements of language tasks that address intercultural goals in medical contexts, and considered some of the issues raised by educational philosophers such as Barnett. We turn now to two sample tasks that illustrate (i) an intercultural approach to language task design in a medical context and (ii) the adaptation of a PBL 'trigger' to allow the kind of critical reflection, and indeed 'understanding,' advocated by intercultural language educators.

# Intercultural Language Tasks for Medical Students: Working with Children

Intercultural language education, as formulated in Byram's *savoirs* for example, has as a curricular goal the ability to 'decentre', and see a situation from the perspective of the other. For example, Byram (1997: 97) states:

> The intercultural speaker knows about the conventions of communication and interaction in their own and the foreign cultures, the unconscious effect of paralinguistic and non-verbal phenomena, alternative explanations of shared concepts, gestures, customs and rituals.

Although Byram tends to express cultural difference in national terms (e.g. 'their own and foreign cultures,') it is elsewhere evident that interculturality more broadly applies to different cultural groups, whether constituted on the grounds of nationality, ethnicity, professional affiliation, gender, social class or age (see above, Chapter 2). Here, we first consider a task that addresses intercultural communication across the divide of age. The task is directed towards those medical professionals who at some point have to interview and treat young children.

Various published guides to medical communication, of course, address this problematic area. The situation is pertinent to intercultural language educators because the guides usually stress the importance of the doctor or nurse adopting the perspective of the child in order to ensure cooperation and to put the child at ease. And, of course, a child's perspective and concerns are usually different from an adult's, as Kohler (1991: 89) observes:

> Inviting the child to describe his problem may not produce such a detailed factual account as you would get from a parent, but his account may emphasize the importance of the condition to the child himself. Whereas a parent may explain that the child has had eczema for a number of years, the child may say 'I have a rash and everyone laughs at me at school.' Children mix with siblings or peers and their reactions have a profound effect on the patient.

Listening to the child and eliciting what the ailment means to him or her is therefore important if the professional wishes to address the patient's concerns directly. Lloyd and Bor (2009) devote a chapter, co-written by Eleftheriadou, to guidelines on communicating with children and young people, and their advice covers management of children, making the physical environment welcoming or comfortable, how to use play and drawings, addressing children and taking histories, paying attention to their feelings, dealing with adolescents, breaking bad news and liaising with parents and other professionals while maintaining confidentiality. As far as language realisations are concerned, they note that professionals may need to perform four general functions with children (adapted from Lloyd & Bor, 2009: 122):

(1) Giving and requesting information (e.g. 'We need to do X so that we can find out about Y.' 'Have you stayed in hospital before?')
(2) Follow up on the implications of the information children supply (e.g. 'You haven't stayed in hospital? What would you like to bring with you?')
(3) Elicit information about relationships (e.g. 'Mummy can stay with you. Who else will you miss?')
(4) Address beliefs and fears (e.g. 'Many people worry about coming to hospital. What will help you worry a little less?')

These kinds of guidelines can be used as the basis of a number of language tasks, which can be devised with reference to the task components discussed above. The intercultural *goal* would be to raise awareness of the child's concerns about the illness as opposed to the parents' or the doctor's. The *input* might be a particular scenario where learners are asked to consider the case of an eight-year-old boy who is presenting with asthma. Learners may be given a brief description of the child's condition, for example:

Datuk is six years old, and has arrived at your clinic with his mother, Fatimah. Both are Malaysian; Datuk's father is studying engineering at the local university.

Datuk has begun to suffer asthma attacks. When these, happen, he finds it difficult to breathe, especially at night, he wheezes and coughs, and his chest is tight.

You are not yet sure what triggers the asthma attacks or how severe they are. Datuk may have been suffering from a respiratory infection, like influenza; he may be allergic to animal pollen; it may be that he has been exercising in cold weather or that he has been exposed to air pollution or tobacco smoke. You might have to recommend a visit to the hospital to do further tests.

The *activity* is to ask learners how they would (a) arrange the doctor's waiting room and surgery to make Dakut, and other children like him, feel comfortable; (b) elicit further information from Dakut and Fatimah; (c) explain Dakut's condition to him directly in simple terms; (d) find out about Dakut's own worries about his condition; and (e) explain to Dakut and his mother what should happen next. Depending on the background knowledge of the learners, this activity might involve the teacher supplying the learners with supplementary, basic information about asthma, possibly downloaded from a reputable health website. Part of the activity would then be 'translating' the health information into plain and simple language so that it is clear to both Dakut and his mother.

The teacher's initial *role* would be to set up the task and observe the learners' attempts to perform the procedures, (a)–(e). The learners' initial role would be to attempt to perform the task, drawing on their current linguistic resources. The *settings* would vary from classroom to classroom: with larger classes, for example, different groups might collaborate on the five activities simultaneously, and then report their decisions back to the whole group; with smaller classes, each activity might be attempted by the whole class in consecutive stages. For each stage, the teacher should be prepared to evaluate and extend the learners' language and ideas; for instance:

(a)   Is the waiting room child friendly? Are there comics to read or toys to play with while waiting? Are the chairs in the surgery appropriate for a small child? How should the doctor dress? Should they explain to the child what each medical instrument (e.g. a stethoscope) is for, before it is used?

(b) What questions would be addressed to Dakut and which to Fatimah? How would they be framed? How would they be phrased? For example, the doctor might say to Dakut, 'I'm just going to check possible reasons why you have started having these attacks. Is there a new pet in the family? Do any of your close friends own pets? At school, do you play sports outside? Do you like playing football?'

(c) The NHS website[1] carries the following information about asthma: *When your child comes into contact with something that irritates their lungs, known as a trigger, their airways become narrow, the lining becomes inflamed, the muscles around them tighten, and there is an increase in the production of sticky mucus or phlegm.* How would the learners rephrase this for Dakut and Fatimah?

(d) What questions might the learners ask Dakut about his own concerns? For example, 'Is it worse during the night or day? How do you feel then? Do the attacks happen at school? Do they frighten the other children?'

(e) How might the learners explain to Dakut about hospital tests and reassure him, for instance by saying that his mother can be present and that he can bring a favourite toy or book with him?

After this period of consolidation and enhancement, the learners can be asked to draw up a list of 'do's and don'ts' about dealing with children, and these may again be compared with similar advice in the published literature (e.g. Lloyd & Bor, 2009: 112). Finally, the teacher can initiate a period of *reflection*, in which learners might be invited to share their own experience and opinions of dealing with children, and whether or not the advice just formulated is realistic in different medical situations – can a clinic in an impoverished country afford toys in the waiting room; can doctors in a busy city practice afford the time to elicit and address a child's concerns? Is it sufficient simply to treat the asthma? Reflection sessions tend to be open-ended; some learners might indeed feel that spending time dealing with a child's concerns *is* an inefficient use of resources. But, as Barnett advises, honest, rational reflection is necessary if the educator is to encourage genuine engagement, rather than simply to pay lip-service to course content. Teachers cannot force the learners to share their views; however, they can present the issues to be addressed and invite the learners to consider and evaluate them from different perspectives.

# Integrating Intercultural Learning with PBL Scenarios

Earlier in this chapter we noted the parallels and some differences between the TBL and PBL models, concluding that the modes of delivery of intercultural language education and medical education were, in many ways, compatible. Indeed Betancourt (2004: 954) advocates PBL specifically as a way of developing cross-cultural competence:

> Interactive, case-based sessions that highlight clinical applications are the ideal methods for teaching cultural competence. When used selectively as the clinical scenario dictates, the skills acquired from such situations can help illuminate the parent's values, beliefs and behavior.

However, we also noted some concern in the literature on PBL that some clinical scenarios focused purely on clinical issues, neglecting the complexities that arise when dealing with 'real world' cases. To counter such concerns, Shields (2008) describes PBL sessions that present case studies of culturally diverse patients presenting with gastrointestinal complaints: an obese woman unable to pay for essential medication; an Asian woman who uses alternative therapies; and a male American war veteran with hepatitis C and alcohol-related liver cirrhosis, who also happens to be addicted to salty bar snacks. In addressing the issues arising from the treatment of different patients with similar ailments, medical students are encouraged to think 'creatively' about the topics of racial, socio-economic and professional biases in favour of or against particular cultural groups, their beliefs and practices. They are invited to consider, for example, whether issues of alternative medicine might only be relevant to Asian patients, and how to influence a patient whose destructive dietary regime is bound up with his socialization and identity (e.g. as a member of a group of relatively hard drinking war veterans).

While, admittedly, little can wholly prepare medical students for the culture shock of clinical practice, PBL sessions can at least attempt to address broader issues with the goal of extending the medical student's intercultural communicative competence. This process may involve adapting existing PBL triggers and refocusing the ensuing discussions. To give a slightly more detailed example from our own experience,[2] a PBL session can be broken down into a complex series of language tasks. Despite its complexity, the task can be broken down into its main constitutive elements. The *goal* would be to encourage medical students to 'decentre' and, this time, consider how advanced age and cultural values might impact on a clinical study. The *input* is a PBL trigger that includes a 78-year-old female Taiwanese patient's complaint, her medical history, the results of a physical examination and lab tests, the initial management and clinical course of treatment, and a list of resources. A summary of the complaint is:

> The patient was accompanied by her son and daughter-in-law to the obstetrics and gynaecology (OBGYN) outpatient clinic with a chief complaint of an excess of red-coloured discharge soaking her underwear about a week ago. Following that incident, she has intermittently been getting dark red discharge on her sanitary pad, which prompted her to revisit the outpatient clinic.

The *procedures* involve a complex problem-solving activity, whereby the learners put forward hypotheses and identify learning issues. The *students' role* in PBL is normally to work in a group *setting* to research, present and discuss possible clinical solutions to a given problem. However, the *teacher's role* in this case is in part to encourage students to identify cultural as well as clinical issues arising from the scenario, and to probe how the students will address them. A potential learning issue arising from the above trigger is to discover the patient's socio-economic or religious background and to elicit how she feels about the discharge – does she, for example, regard it as 'unclean'? Some research into the beliefs and attitudes of communities to menstruation might be suggested. The students might consider doing further research into how to communicate with patients about symptoms that they might consider embarrassing or distasteful. Sometimes patients with symptoms they find embarrassing are silent when questioned. Clare (1991: 23) suggests that in such cases:

> The doctor may break the silence by repeating the last question or indeed the patient's last response or by indicating that perhaps the patient feels anxious or shy or a little fearful of talking further. Acknowledging that it can in certain circumstances be difficult to put things into words often helps ease the situation for the patient.

In this particular PBL, students are given information that is explicitly related to common cultural attitudes among elderly Taiwanese females. In an interview, a gynaecologist in the same institution indicated to us that such females are often 'reserved' and resist having procedures that they consider intrusive, such as pap tests. Since the medical students have to understand the need for more extensive explanation and reassurance in such cases, an extension to the scenario was added: 'The doctor asks if the patient has done the pap test. Ms Wu [the daughter-in-law] replied that the patient would feel too embarrassed to do this test at such a late age'. As with Shields' case studies, the students then have to consider what impact the patient's beliefs and attitudes might have on how they would treat her, and what explanation they would give to her about her treatment.

Of course one point about PBL outcomes is that they are not predictable. The facilitator might hint to the students that they are neglecting the cultural circumstances of the patient, whom they might see simply as a clinical problem to be solved. A period of *reflection* is therefore again necessary to match the PBL tutorial outcomes against the initial goals set by the designers of the curriculum and the PBL tasks. If students have missed cues that attention to attitudes, beliefs and cultural behaviour is important, this neglect can be addressed then. If the students have paid attention to these cues, their understanding can be tested through further discussion: for example, do they really believe it is necessary to spend valuable time on concerns about a patient's embarrassment?

In short, the assumption underpinning PBL is that the intercultural speaker's competence is acquired not from an exposure to an inventory or checklist of necessary skills, or even from involvement in 'thin' managed simulations, with simple and predictable outcomes sanctioned by the teacher. Rather skilled practitioners are developed from an exposure to rich, immersive experiences that are closely modelled on real-life situations. PBL comprises a complex set of language tasks that present learners with numerous challenges, particularly when the activities demand behaviour – such as challenging tutors – that learners find culturally unfamiliar. However, when conducted imaginatively, PBL offers a rich way of addressing intercultural issues in medicine and encouraging learners to engage in 'intercultural being'.

This chapter and the previous one have given an overview of some of the issues that arise when intercultural language education is combined with medical education. The previous chapter considered the correspondence in the educational agenda of intercultural language teachers and those of medical educators interested in developing cross-cultural competences. In the present chapter, we have looked at task-based practices that can be used in the teaching and learning of intercultural language skills in a medical context. The following chapters will open out some of these issues in greater detail, and add others. Chapters 4 and 5 focus on developing linguistic competences, which are still a central component of intercultural communicative competence. Chapter 6 revisits critical cultural awareness in medical contexts; Chapters 7 and 8 consider the role of the medical humanities in addressing issues of language and values; and Chapter 9 considers the question of course design, before the concluding chapter summarises the issues raised by this volume as a whole.

## Notes

(1) http://www.nhs.uk/Conditions/Asthma-in-children/Pages/Introduction.aspx Accessed 27 May 2011.
(2) The scenario is adapted with permission from a script originally written in Chinese by Dr Te-Fu Chan of Kaohsiung Medical University, and then translated into English by Peih-ying Lu for use by KMU students whose medical programme was being delivered through the medium of English.

# 4 Exploring Medical Language

The move towards an intercultural approach to teaching English in medical education does not mean that concerns with the distinctive nature of medical language should be ignored or neglected. Indeed, in formulations of intercultural language education, theorists restate the fundamental importance of what Byram (1997: 10) calls 'linguistic competence' (e.g. Byram, 1997: 10, 16) and Risager calls 'languastructural competence' (e.g. Risager, 2007: 227). While arguing that earlier curricular models used by language educators focused too much on knowledge of the phonology, grammar and vocabulary of the target medium, at the expense of non-linguistic features (which Byram formulates as the *savoirs*; see Chapter 2), Byram and Risager nevertheless agree that knowledge of the structural resources of the language is a desirable goal amongst learners. Part of an intercultural language curriculum in a medical context, then, may still legitimately be devoted to tasks that focus on developing learners' awareness of the linguistic nature of medical language. The present chapter, therefore, focuses broadly on medical language while Chapter 5 turns to the key issue of face-to-face interactions in a range of medical contexts.

The nature of medical language is itself, of course, a substantial topic to address. The academic study of specialised language and its application to language teaching was given impetus by the development of 'register analysis' in the 1960s (e.g. Halliday *et al.*, 1964) and 'genre analysis' in the 1980s and 1990s (e.g. Swales, 1990; Nwogu, 1997). Since then there have been various studies of the nature of written and spoken language as it is used in medical contexts. To name only a few, Atkinson (1992), Williams (1996) and Taavitsainen and Pahta (2011) all offer different perspectives on medical writing in historical and contemporary periods, while Maher (1986) traces the development of English as an international language of medicine. Much scholarly and pedagogical attention has focused on the differences between medical text types (e.g. Biber & Finegan, 1994) and the evolving and dynamic differences between the technical registers of medical professionals and 'everyday' discourse of non-professionals (Nwogu, 1991; Nwogu & Bloor, 1991). The 'everyday versus professional' distinction is important in medical education for two reasons: first, medical students are developing the technical language necessary to communicate with fellow-professionals; second, as they develop their professional, technical medical registers, students nevertheless need to maintain an awareness of the cultural divide between professional and non-professional discourses. Medical students need to acquire a sensitive flexibility in using appropriate language – professional or everyday – depending on the audience and purpose of their discourse. Language learning tasks, then, may be directed towards addressing the 'everyday culture' of non-professional medical discourse versus the 'professional culture' of peer-directed medical discourse.

The present chapter considers how digital resources may be used to devise tasks that explore the tension between lay and professional discourses. We argue that digital resources offer a rich and varied means of analysing the use of medical language by non-professionals and professionals alike. Like most other disciplines, medicine, linguistics and language education have all been affected by the revolution in information technology over the past few decades. Whereas in the not-so-distant past, some families might have owned a copy of a large, thick medical encyclopaedia, now many people with a health complaint can access advice online, either at home or through a library. Healthcare professionals, too, have instant access to medical databases and electronic journals. The democratisation of access to health-care advice online has changed the nature of face-to-face doctor-patient interaction. In our experience, doctors sometimes complain that patients present at their clinics not only with symptoms but with a ready, though not always reliable, diagnosis. The availability of online medical information raises issues of expertise and authority that is further complicated by the call, in many healthcare contexts, for 'patient-centred' medical practices.

Language education too has been – and continues to be – radically transformed by the proliferation of digital resources. The description of language, particularly spoken language, has been enriched by the availability of collections of searchable, digitised texts: most pedagogical dictionaries and grammar books now make a virtue of being corpus-based, and many are available online, accessible by both computer and mobile phone. Most language teachers also have a wealth of textual and visual data, medical and general, available at the touch of a keyboard. Materials design and classroom pedagogy have been slower to respond to the digital revolution, but guides like Aijmer (2009), Anderson and Corbett (2009), Bennett (2010), Hunston (2002) and O'Keeffe et al. (2007) have demonstrated how teachers might embed insights from corpus linguistics in the language classroom. The present chapter, then, takes one particular approach to the ways in which language teachers in medical contexts might encourage learners to explore the technical and everyday registers of medicine. We focus here on tasks that use digital resources to explore aspects of technical and everyday language in medicine. For example, reliable healthcare portals are a rich source of medical language, and tools for electronic text analysis can be used in conjunction with these digital resources to shed light on aspects of medical language. But digital resources can also be used in intercultural language classrooms to go beyond 'linguistic competence': teachers can devise tasks that raise issues of cultural preconceptions, ethics and authority, and to explore how certain groups in society construct images of themselves and discuss their health issues. Accordingly, the present chapter will consider:

- Healthcare websites as a source of medical language and content.
- Specialised medical corpora and general corpora (Teenage Healthfreak; Patientvoices; Healthtalkonline; TIME, BNC, CoCA).
- How to use corpora and text-analysis tools to analyse medical discourse.

# Healthcare Portals as a Source of Medical Language and Content

There are many websites that act as portals for a range of information on healthcare, and here we mention only an illustrative few.[1] Some sites, such as Healthlinks.net, based in the USA, and Aarogya.com in India are commercial services which seek to act as a healthcare portal, to collate and provide comprehensive and reliable information on many aspects of healthcare issues for use by members of the public and by professionals. Teachers using them should, however, note that while they claim to monitor and vet all content that can be accessed via the portal, they cannot take legal responsibility for errors or inaccuracy in the information they link to. Healthlink. net's directory of information covers the alphabet from alternative health, including acupuncture and massage, to veterinary medicine and women's health. There is a newsletter on healthcare issues, ranging from a case report on HIV/AIDS in older patients to advice for professionals on how to 'live with your mistakes'. Teachers of medical language should also find the audio-visual library of short presentations useful: topics currently covered include healthy eating, hypertension, migraines, prostate cancer and 'true stories'. Finally, users can register to participate in a forum whereby they can seek and give information and support on a variety of health issues. Similarly, Aarogya provides information in three languages to those in need of health advice, and also describes itself as 'ideally suited as a tool for brand building.' Among other sources of general information is Wikipedia's 'Health and Fitness' portal.

State-run websites vary in their function: the American healthcare.gov website mainly collates information on private and public medical insurance options for US citizens, while the Australian Health*insite* and the UK's NHS Direct aim to supplement face-to-face and telephone services by including encyclopaedic information, and further features, such as chatrooms and (in the case of NHS Direct) an interactive symptom-checker. Like the Healthlinks.net website, NHS Direct is at pains to emphasise the limitations of web-based inquiry, noting that the information given is not intended to replace a consultation with a qualified professional. The development of the Australian Health*insite* portal, however, was a direct response to the challenge of controlling the quality of healthcare advice on the web, in an environment in which more and more people are turning to the internet for advice:

> In line with the Australian Government's strategy of delivering services via the Internet by 2001, Health*Insite* was conceived to bridge the gap between the increasing potential for consumers to access health information via the Internet, and the absence of quality control of web information.

Without doubt one of the attractions of the internet for 'consumers' is that it allows them to seek health advice without the intimidating, embarrassing or otherwise threatening face-to-face presence of a doctor. Several websites have been set up to support people seeking advice who are having difficulty coming to terms with their illness, or who want to reach out to others experiencing the same symptoms and side effects. The charity website, Patientvoices, is a resource that currently makes available over 100 digitised stories about healthcare; it is designed for use by patients and healthcare providers, and has been used in the UK for medical education. It is a valuable source of spoken material; however, there are at present no transcripts available of the spoken testimonies, a fact that makes the resource more difficult to use in language education. There are, however, related educational resources downloadable from the website.

Healthtalkonline, similarly, was started by two doctors on a charitable basis; it currently provides interviews and written testimony of around 2000 people's experiences of illness and healthcare. For example, at the time of writing, the resource made available 26 interviews with members of ethnic minority communities who were caring for family members with mental health issues. Several of these interviews are in minority languages, including Cantonese and Gujerati. The audio-visual interviews are given alongside a written verbatim transcript that is extremely useful to language educators, as we shall demonstrate below.

Some web-based resources target precisely those members of the community who are less likely to seek a face-to-face appointment with an authority-figure. For example, the Healthtalkonline resource has a facility aimed at younger patients (www.youthealthtalk.org), and the 'Teenage Health Freak' website is another interactive resource established by doctors with the mission to give 'cringe-free' advice to teenagers. The homepage features the generic 'Dr Ann' answering questions such as, 'What is cocaine?' 'Am I overweight?' and 'When is the right age to have sex?' Many current healthcare websites acknowledge the fast-changing nature of medical knowledge. The sites are regularly updated, and, as web technology also evolves, the ways in which users interact with the websites also change. As a consequence, the illustrative sites and online services used in this chapter are subject to continual updating; therefore, we focus here on general principles involved in using digital resources rather than specific issues arising from the use of any particular content.

## Exploring Medical Language with Online Resources

Any teacher who enjoys internet access can make use of electronic text analysis tools to explore many aspects of medical language with their learners. At one level, web resources offer a set of texts that are rich in medical content and directed at different audiences: patients, professionals and trainees. Teachers of medical language can simply select from these sites texts that expose learners to relevant vocabulary items and afford insights into their 'authentic' use. Teachers and learners who further develop their skills in electronic text analysis can also exploit online resources to teach themselves more about the nature of medical discourse.

Most text analysis tools currently available focus on four features of lexical usage:

(a)  how frequently a word (or search item, or node) appears in a text;
(b)  the words most closely associated with the search item (its collocates);
(c)  how the node appears in a short sequence of text (its concordance line);
(d)  whether or not the presence of a search item is 'key' in a given text (i.e. whether it appears either unusually frequently or unusually infrequently in that text).

For further, more general advice on exploring English with online digital resources, see Anderson and Corbett (2009), and for illustrative case studies using other small corpora, see Bondi *et al.* (2004). Some corpus-informed studies have been undertaken on medical language; see, for example, Carter, Skelton, Kenkre and Hobbs' (1997) discussion of aggressive language in the medical workplace, Skelton, Murray and Hobbs' (1999) analysis of 'imprecision' in consultations between a consultant hematologist and seriously ill patients, and Ferguson's (2001) study of the use of 'if conditionals' in medical discourse. For a more specific example, we first consider the analysis of a corpus designed to give teenagers medical advice, and then consider how to build and analyse customised corpora for our own use.

# Medical Terms in General Corpora: Frequency and Collocation

As educators, we can use the internet to make our own specialised corpora, or we can pay attention to the insights gained from others' analysis of corpora of medical interactions (see below). Most immediately, however, teachers and students can exploit large corpora of general and specialised language for the light they shed on medical language and cultural concerns. In this section we demonstrate some simple ways of using the following freely-accessible online corpora, mainly compiled or made available by Mark Davies of Brigham Young University[2]:

- The Corpus of Contemporary American English (CoCA): currently 425 million words of text from a range of sources such as fiction, newspapers, magazines, academic and unscripted broadcast speech.
- The British National Corpus (BNC): 100 million words of text from a similar range of written sources, as well as recorded and transcribed casual speech.
- The TIME corpus: 100 million words from *Time* magazine, selected from the 1920s to the 2000s. This last corpus is useful as a source of changing journalistic attitudes to a range of subjects, including medicine and health, over almost a century.

The availability and easy use of these large-scale corpora allows educators and language learners to deal with large amounts of language in a few seconds, identify language patterns, learn how words are used in a range of written and spoken contexts, and identify cultural 'hotspots' and 'shifts'. Learners can also use the corpora to extend the range of their own linguistic repertoire.

To take a simple example of a language pattern, CoCA and BNC can be searched to identify the most common adjectives that pre-modify 'cough' in American and British English. To do this, we can search the corpora for any kind of adjective [j*] plus the noun 'cough'.

---

## Activity: Searching for frequently used adjectives

(1) Go to http://corpus.byu.edu/coca.
(2) Click on 'List'.
(3) Type your search item: [j*] cough.
(4) Click 'Search'.

---

This will give you a list of the most frequently used adjectives with 'cough' in the corpus. If you then click 'Compare Results: BNC' at the top of the screen, then you can compare the American results with the British corpus. At the present time, the top 10 results are shown in Table 4.1.

The results show that 'cough' is modified by a wide range of adjectives; however, learners might familiarise themselves with the most frequently used. The two corpora suggest that four adjectives occur frequently across the two corpora: *persistent, dry, little* and *bad*. Teachers familiarising learners with different ways of describing coughs might encourage them to group

**Table 4.1** Top frequencies of [ADJECTIVE] + cough in CoCA and BNC

| CoCA | Frequency (per 425 million) | BNC | Frequency (per 100 million) |
|---|---|---|---|
| Chronic cough | 66 | Dry cough | 19 |
| Persistent cough | 38 | Productive cough | 9 |
| Dry cough | 31 | Persistent cough | 8 |
| Little cough | 24 | Little cough | 8 |
| Bad cough | 20 | Barking cough | 7 |
| Over-the-counter cough | 18 | Bad cough | 7 |
| Deep cough | 15 | Slight cough | 6 |
| Small cough | 9 | Rasping cough | 5 |
| Productive cough | 8 | Nasty cough | 5 |
| Slight cough | 8 | Spasmodic cough | 4 |

those adjectives that express the extent of the cough (*little, small, slight* versus *bad, nasty*), those that express its frequency (*chronic, persistent, spasmodic*), those that describe the sound it makes (*deep, barking, rasping*), and those that say whether or not it is accompanied by phlegm (*dry* versus *productive*). There are two apparent differences between the two corpora: the high frequency in CoCA of *chronic cough* and the presence, in the same corpus, of the apparently anomalous *over-the-counter cough*.

To investigate these two phrases further, re-do the search of CoCA, but this time click 'Chart' rather than 'List', and type *chronic cough* and *over-the-counter cough* as your search items. This will show you the genres in which the terms occur, and larger contexts for the phrases will be given in the results. These searches show that in CoCA *chronic cough* occurs by far the most frequently in academic, or professional, written texts; it is not used very frequently in non-academic, or everyday, genres. Its relative infrequency in the BNC data may be a consequence of different sampling strategies for academic texts. Moreover, *over-the-counter* is part of a fuller phrase, namely *over-the-counter cough medicine*, an expression most frequently found in magazine data in the period 2005–2008. It is further evident from a closer examination of the results, that a report on this topic was published in 2007, and the relative frequency of the phrase in the American data is again probably because many of the CoCA samples are taken from a range of print and broadcast media.

The teacher of English to medical students will no doubt be able to imagine a range of ways in which online corpora can be used to teach the specialised vocabulary of the discipline. To take another brief example, teachers of medical vocabulary often focus on the etymological roots of words as ways of grouping related technical terms: the prefix *gastr(o)*, for example, refers to the stomach while *cardi(o)* refers to the heart. A search for the 10 most frequent words beginning with *gastr(o)* in CoCA can be performed easily by redoing the search described above, but using as the search item the wildcard *gastr\** to cover all the lexical items beginning with the letters $g + a + s + t + r$. The results of the search identify eight words that are largely medical and two that belong to a different domain – which itself makes a useful 'odd one out' activity (see Table 4.2).

If the learners are having difficulty in identifying the two 'non-medical' terms in this list, they can be encouraged to do a 'key word in context' search on each item, which will show that the third and sixth on the list above appear in such phrases as 'pure gastronomic bliss', which are clearly to do with the culinary and not the medical domain.

Large online corpora of general language can be used to demonstrate both everyday and professional uses of medical terminology. Journalistic

**Table 4.2** Highest frequencies for *gastr\** as a search item in CoCA

| Term | Frequency |
| --- | --- |
| 1. Gastrointestinal | 855 |
| 2. Gastric | 502 |
| 3. Gastronomic | 173 |
| 4. Gastroenteritis | 145 |
| 5. Gastroenterologist | 124 |
| 6. Gastronomy | 84 |
| 7. Gastroenterology | 77 |
| 8. Gastroesophageal | 74 |
| 9. Gastritis | 58 |
| 10. Gastroenterologists | 52 |

corpora, like TIME, can equally be used to explore popular attitudes towards medical issues. For example, to explore the distribution of words related to contraception over the decades from the 1920s to the 2000s, teachers can do the following search. This time the wild-card *contracept\** is used to find related words like *contraception(s), contraceptive(s)*, and so on. The 'Chart' search in the TIME corpus does not list the highest frequency items; instead it displays the number of occurrences in the text samples, decade by decade (Figure 4.1).

## Activity: Tracking word frequencies through time

(1) Go to http://corpus.byu.edu/time.
(2) Click on 'Chart'.
(3) Type your search item: contracept\*.
(4) Click 'Search'.

The results will look something like Figure 4.1. The results suggest that there was a surge in the reporting of contraception as a topic in the 1960s in *Time* magazine, and that the reporting of contraception has stayed relatively higher after that decade than it was beforehand. The reasons for this are not hard to find: the contraceptive pill began to be produced in the 1960s, and this heralded a major cultural shift in popular attitudes to birth control and sexual behaviour.

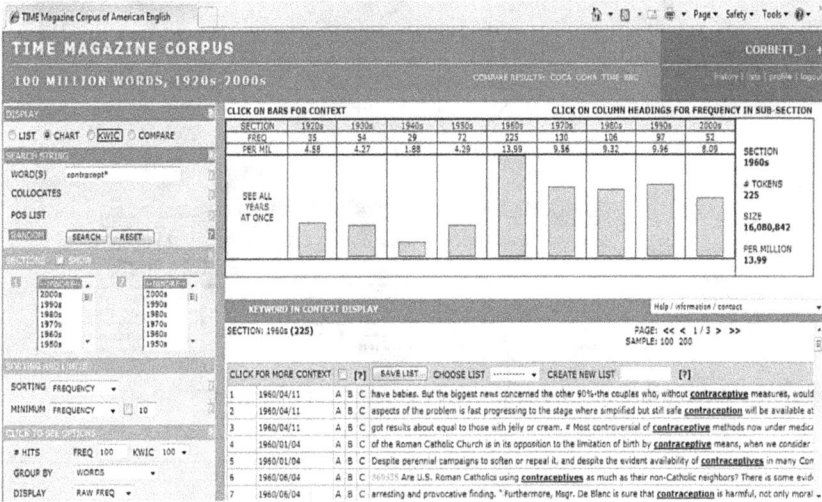

**Figure 4.1** Screenshot of CoCA search for *contracept** decade-by-decade

The frequency results, decade by decade, are a visible indicator of the cultural impact of this medical innovation; to explore it further we can search the corpus to identify the collocates of *contracept**, that is, those co-occurring words most strongly 'tied' to the search item by reason of frequency and mutual presence. Corpora like CoCA allow us to identify collocates by assigning them a score arrived at by a statistical operation known as the calculation of 'Mutual Information' (MI). Mutual Information takes into account the frequency of co-occurrence of two items and also whether the items commonly co-occur with other terms. For example, we can guess that since the 1960s, at least, 'contraceptive' has co-occured frequently with 'pill', to the extent that 'The Pill' has become synonymous with contraceptive pills. We would therefore expect a search for collocates of *contracept** to give 'pill' a high MI score. But 'contraceptive' might also collocate with other words, including grammatical items like 'and', which co-occur with many different words. Unless there is an abnormally high co-occurrence of 'and' and *contracept**, then, we would expect a grammatical term like 'and' to have a lower MI score than 'pill' since it is not so uniquely 'bound' to the search item. Conventionally, an MI score that is higher than three indicates a statistically significant bond between two collocates; the higher the score, the stronger the bond. The top 20 collocates of *contracept** in the TIME corpus as a whole are shown in Figure 4.2.

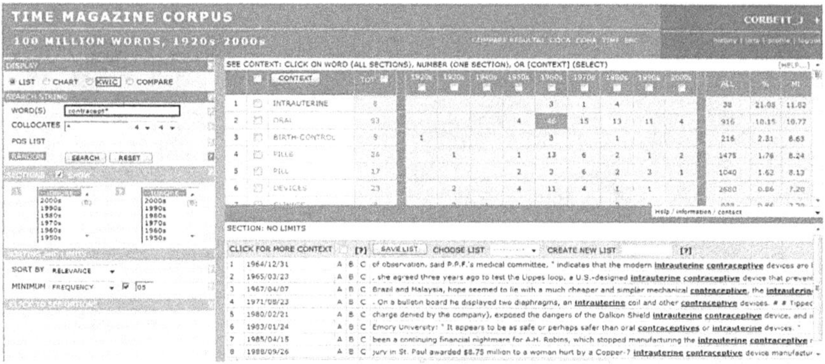

**Figure 4.2** Screenshot of TIME search for collocates of *contracept**

---

## Activity: Searching for collocates

(1)  Go to http://corpus.byu.edu/time.
(2)  Click on 'List'.
(3)  Type your search item: contracept*.
(4)  Click 'Collocate' and keep the span of words as four on each side. Leave the Collocate search box empty for the time being (if you wish, you can search for collocates that are verbs, nouns, adjectives, etc.).
(5)  In the 'Sorting and Limits' section, set 'Sort by' to 'Relevance' and the minimum frequency to 'five'.
(6)  Click 'Search'.

---

The top 20 collocates of *contracept** in the TIME corpus, sorted by relevance (that is, by MI score) but with the frequency also shown, are given in Table 4.3.

The first two collocates, *intrauterine* and *oral* show the difference between simple frequency of co-occurrence and the measurement of Mutual Information. While *intrauterine* only occurs with *contracept** eight times, there is a particularly strong bond insofar as most or all of these occurrences will be within a four-word span to either side of the search item. *Oral*, on the other hand, very frequently co-occurs with *contracept** (93 times) but it will co-occur with a number of other words too (e.g. *oral hygiene*), and so the 'tie' is calculated to be slightly weaker. To filter out the particularly rare words that might occur only a few times in the corpus, near *contracept**, a minimum frequency was set of five occurrences. Re-sorting the list by frequency of

**Table 4.3** Top 20 collocates of *contracept\** in TIME, sorted according to MI score

| Collocates 1-10 | MI Score | Freq. | Collocates 11-20 | MI Score | Freq. |
|---|---|---|---|---|---|
| intrauterine | 11.82 | 8 | prescription | 6.49 | 6 |
| oral | 10.77 | 93 | methods | 6.12 | 19 |
| birth-control | 8.63 | 5 | barrier | 6.07 | 5 |
| pills | 8.24 | 26 | couples | 5.90 | 7 |
| pill | 8.13 | 17 | forbidden | 5.58 | 6 |
| devices | 7.20 | 23 | device | 5.40 | 9 |
| clinics | 7.20 | 8 | distribution | 5.27 | 5 |
| abortion | 6.88 | 20 | Catholics | 5.25 | 9 |
| unmarried | 6.81 | 5 | method | 5.17 | 10 |
| artificial | 6.53 | 13 | emergency | 5.16 | 12 |

occurrence would show a more general vocabulary related to the search item, which is sometimes useful.

What we see in Table 4.3, then, is effectively a 'cultural profile' of the way the words related to *contraception* are used an American magazine, based on those words that are most strongly 'tied' to the search item, *contracept\**. Again, the words can usefully be grouped into categories (some of which may overlap):

- General procedures: *birth-control, device(s), method(s), artificial.*
- Specific procedures and places: *intrauterine, oral, pill(s), barrier, clinics, pre-scription, emergency.*
- Personal and moral issues: *couples, forbidden, unmarried, abortion, catholics.*

This grouping can be used as the basis for discussion of the popular reception of this form of medical provision historically – the results further break the frequencies of co-occurrence down decade by decade, so, for example we can see at a glance that 'oral' occurs very frequently in the 1960s while 'information', 'advice' and 'methods' occur relatively frequently in the 1920s and 1930s.

A large and carefully designed corpus like TIME can provide teachers and students with much linguistic evidence for the popular perception of medical issues; however it is worth recalling that corpora can only give information about what is written and talked about. Searches for instances of *breast cancer* show very few results until the rise of feminism and the public discussion of a broader range of women's concerns (the frequency rises gradually from one in the 1920s to 17 in the 1960s, and then jumps to 83 in the 1970s). A similar pattern is seen for *testicular cancer*, which is simply not mentioned until the 1970s and is relatively rarely discussed in the popular press even now. For more substantial data on focused topics, we need to turn to more specialised 'medical' corpora.

## Insights from a Medical Corpus: Teenage Health Freak

A fascinating example of the compilation and analysis of a specific medical resource is the corpus of 1 million words compiled of emails sent to the British adolescent health website Teenage Health Freak (http://www.teenagehealthfreak.org). This corpus was designed to explore adolescents' use of language in relation to the often vexed topic of their health, a topic that they regularly have difficulty in communicating to adults, particularly authority figures such as parents and doctors. A subset of this corpus of emails (roughly 400,000 words) has been widely discussed, for example in Adolphs *et al.* (2004), Brown *et al.* (2006: 130–139), Brown *et al.* (2008), Harvey *et al.* (2007) and Crawford and Brown (2010). Adolescents' anonymous emails to 'Dr Ann', the 'virtual doctor' who gives advice on the website are, as the corpus compilers claim, useful sources of current 'everyday, colloquial expressions of patients' ailments' (Crawford & Brown, 2010: 6) and an intriguing index of teenagers' particular health concerns and anxieties.

The kinds of analysis performed on the Teenage Health Freak corpus mirrors, on a larger scale, those illustrated earlier in this chapter: frequency analysis and comparison between medical and more general corpora, in this case CANCODE, the corpus of general spoken English. An analysis of the frequency of vocabulary items used in the Teenage Health Freak corpus reveals, for example, teenagers' particular concern with issues of sexuality (Harvey *et al.*, 2007: 774). What is particularly interesting is the frequency of terms related to sexual health, which significantly exceeds the frequency we would expect in a corpus such as TIME, CoCA or the BNC. Although the website solicits input across a whole range of health issues, it is sexuality and reproductive health that predominate in the emails, inasmuch as terms like 'penis', 'pregnant', 'period' and 'gay' feature far more frequently than they do in non-medical corpora. A related issue that proved to be a particular concern for adolescents was their perceived normalcy. Having noted that 'normal' appears with an unusual degree of frequency (or a high degree of 'keyness'; see further below) in the Teenage Health Freak corpus, the analysts proceeded to a finer-grained analysis of concordance lines, which

(1) I'm 12, I'm 5, 3 ft and 42 kg is this a **normal** weight or is it too light?
(2) or being flat chested. Worried boobs aren't **normal** size. episodes of Bulimia
(3) seen that is **normal**. But I dont want to b **normal** I want to be thin. I find it insulting
(4) 14 and I havent started my period am I **normal** I masterbate. I use
(5) sick for no apparant reason. Is it **normal** to miss a period for 3 months
(6) thinking about becoming a transexual. Is it **normal** to do this?
(7) been a little depressed recently. Is this **normal** ?
(8) ward and I havent got any pubic hair am I **normal** ?. I am 13 and my name
(9) this white stuff in my under wear, am I **normal** or do I have a disease.
(10) is phone sex **normal** because I've had it a couple of times with 2 boys

**Figure 4.3** Selected concordance lines for 'normal', adapted from Harvey *et al.* (2007: 776); see also Crawford and Brown (2010: 12)

showed the use of the search item, 'normal' in a range of contexts. Some of these are reproduced in Figure 4.3.

As Harvey *et al.* (2007) and Crawford and Brown (2010) observe, the corpus, in bringing together a range of uses of the term 'normal,' illuminates its idiomatic senses, which go beyond the idea that something may or may not be statistically 'average.' While seeking advice on a range of norms relating to sexual and mental health, teenagers are also seeking information about cultural identity. As Crawford and Brown (2010: 12) put it:

In his work on discipline, regulation and the production of social and scientific order, Foucault (eg 1979, 1980) described what he called 'normalising practises' where particular sets of behaviours are learned and regulated through a process of comparison. There are a variety of disciplines that may be involved in the process of normalisation, for example, education, professional training, the hospital system and various other systems that are capable of setting normative standards for health and wellbeing.

Teenagers, at a crucial phase in their process of self-formation, are using healthcare advice in part to monitor their experience against a set of normative standards as expressed by the 'virtual' doctor, Dr Ann. They are also evaluating aspects of their own physicality (e.g. weight, breast size, growth of pubic hair) against a culturally constructed set of idealised 'norms', conformity to which would allow them as individuals to 'fit in' or even excel as part of their peer group. 'Normal' in this case does not simply mean 'statistically average' but also, effectively, 'desirable' in the context of a perceived deviation, whether this is through absence, insufficiency or excess.

Corpus analysis of a relatively large number of healthcare interactions, then, can identify how people articulate health issues, and also how their construction of social reality, including their self-image, is achieved partly through discursive engagement on the topic of health with peers and professionals. It can indicate areas of particular concern, like sexual health. Doctors who are dealing with adolescents, at least in the UK, which is the main source of the Teenage Health Freak corpus, may be trained to be alert to words like 'normal' as indicating the patient's anxious sense of his or her possible deviation from an idealised and desirable norm. The question then arises – can language teachers and learners adapt the techniques used by the Teenage Health Freak researchers to inform their own understanding of how people use language in medical contexts?

## Data Collection: Everyday Perspectives on Mental Health Care

There are, as noted above, many websites devoted to medical issues. One possibility for teachers interested in working with learners to explore medical 'languastructure' is to build up your own digital corpus of medical texts from the sources available on the web, and to do some basic linguistic analyses using text-analysis software that, at the time of writing, is freely available.[3] The example chosen here for illustrative purposes is a section of www.healthtalkonline.org that contains interviews with a selection of people from ethnic communities who are caring for family members with mental health problems. The transcripts that have been made available are reasonably brief and cover a range of positions on mental health care from different personal and cultural perspectives; for example, here is the view of 'Tina', an Asian woman in her late 50s, who is caring for a son and working in a community centre:

> Rather than forcing you should give them treatment, if the person doesn't take treatment you should give something in the water or in the food, and that way you can find out the 'cureness'. But if they say that, we should, the law is very bad for this country. When the person has a mental balance then they don't say or hesitate taking the medication, but

this kind of schizophrenia or any mental depression or many mental illness, the doctor should give the treatment in food or any available drink, when they refuse it they should do like that and cure the person. This is my personal opinion. (http://www.healthtalkonline.org/mental_health/mentalhealthcarers/People/Interview/1774/Category/334)

The transcript reproduces some of the features of everyday spoken discourse – the loose, grammatical structures and the creativity in spontaneously creating new words, like 'cureness'. There are also indications that the speaker is a non-native, given constructions such as *rather than forcing you should give them treatment* where a native speaker might say something like 'instead of forcing treatment on them'. The carer's view is nevertheless clearly expressed, and serves as an opinion that might provoke discussion on topics such as the rights of patients whose sense of personal responsibility might be diminished. It is, however, as the carer acknowledges, 'a personal view'. A corpus-based study can incorporate a text like this with other texts from similar sources – here mental health carers from ethnic communities – and look quantitatively at trends in their language use. This kind of text analysis opens the possibility of extending the analysis to embrace a broader picture of carers' concerns.

To exemplify the procedure, we have downloaded and saved seven of the transcripts as plain-text files, identified by the given names of the carer, that is, 'Tina', 'Nick', 'Guo', 'Anton 1 and 2', 'Amar' and 'Aiko'. This gives a small but coherent corpus of 4,423 words. It is obviously too small a corpus to be taken as representative, even of the discourse of carers from ethnic communities – but that it not its purpose. The following analysis is largely in the service of a pedagogical exploration of the cultural topics and themes that this particular set of texts represents.

## Analysing frequencies

There are various ways in which teachers and medical students can consider the data contained in a small corpus of texts like the 'carers' corpus'. Here the simple text-analysis software AntConc is used to demonstrate different types of analysis. The first simple, but relatively unrevealing, approach is to look at the frequency of individual lexical items. Extracts from seven carers' transcripts can be loaded into AntConc and the frequencies of the individual grammatical and lexical items can easily be shown (Figure 4.4). The top 30 items of this corpus are shown in Table 4.4.

The results of a search for the most frequently used items in the 'carers' corpus' show that it conforms to the expectations of spoken discourse.

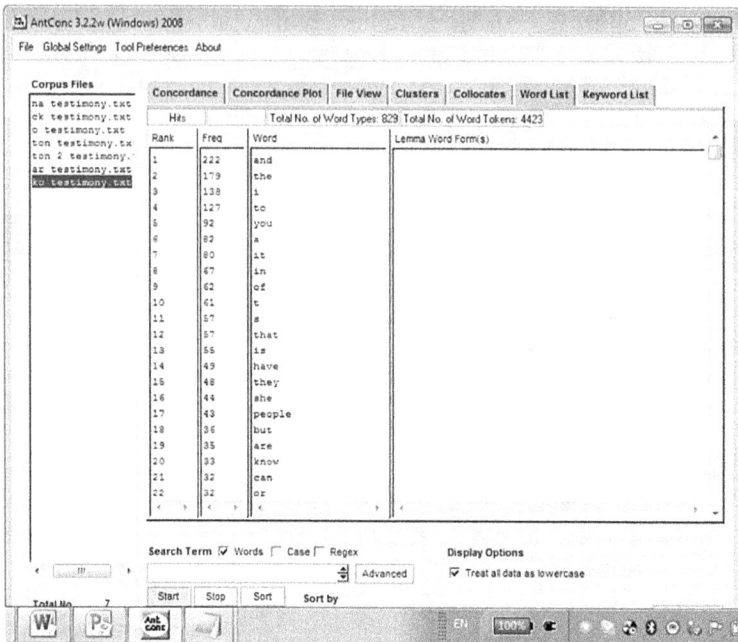

**Figure 4.4** Vocabulary items in the 'carers' corpus' sorted by frequency using AntConc

A comparison of the 'carers' corpus' with the much larger Cambridge and Nottingham Corpus of Discourse in English (CANCODE) reveals that the most frequently used items are largely closed class grammatical items (i.e. pronouns, conjunctions, prepositions, auxiliary verbs) and often-used lexical items like forms of the copula 'be' and the verb 'have'. Writing about the

**Table 4.4** The most frequent items in the 'carers' corpus'

| 1 and | 11 's | 21 can |
|-------|--------|---------|
| 2 the | 12 that | 22 or |
| 3 I | 13 is | 23 so |
| 4 to | 14 have | 24 was |
| 5 you | 15 they | 25 my |
| 6 a | 16 she | 26 then |
| 7 it | 17 people | 27 me |
| 8 in | 18 but | 28 on |
| 9 of | 19 are | 29 there |
| 10 't | 20 know | 30 we |

nature of such items in spoken discourse, O'Keeffe *et al.* (2007: 36) note that the high frequency of pronouns and discourse markers suggests that speakers use them for the purpose of:

projecting their self image, creating good relations with their interlocutors, understanding and using the basic grammatical and logical relations that underpin the less frequent vocabulary.

Table 4.5 demonstrates how even the small 'carers' corpus' largely reproduces the frequency patterns found in CANCODE.

Of particular note are the frequencies of 'I' and 'you', the pronouns that acknowledge the 'here-and-now' of the speech situation. The only lexical item in the 'top 20' in the carers' corpus, alongside the general term, 'people', is 'know', but as O'Keeffe *et al.* also point out, its frequency in speech is largely to do with its use in the complex discourse marker 'you know', which raises common ground between speaker and hearer, and invites a shared perspective on the propositions being expressed.

Even in topic-based language such as mental health, then, the most frequently occurring items are everyday grammatical and logical items that generally organise the concepts being expressed. This is an important point to recall: much of so-called 'specialised' discourse still makes use of a fairly limited set of frequently occurring grammatical and discursive features. However, a legitimate question to ask of any text or set of texts is whether any items occur with an *unusually* high or low frequency. In the case of the carers' corpus, for example, which terms occur more or less frequently compared with their occurrence in other kinds of discourse? The answer to this

**Table 4.5** Comparison of high-frequency items in the 'carers' corpus' and CANCODE

| Carers | CANCODE | Carers | CANCODE |
|--------|---------|--------|---------|
| 1 and | the | 11 's | in |
| 2 the | and | 12 that | was |
| 3 I | I | 13 is | it's |
| 4 to | you | 14 have | know |
| 5 you | it | 15 they | is |
| 6 a | to | 16 she | mm |
| 7 it | a | 17 people | er |
| 8 in | yeah | 18 but | but |
| 9 of | that | 19 are | so |
| 10 't | of | 20 know | they |

question potentially can give a kind of 'semantic profile' of a text, indicating what lexis is privileged or not preferred.

## Analysing Key Words to Show Salience

One way of analysing lexical salience in a set of texts is keyword analysis (e.g. Baker, 2006: 121–152). Keyword analysis is a statistical measure of whether certain expressions appear with unusually high or low frequency in a set of data, compared with a larger 'reference corpus' and it was used to demonstrate, for example, that sexual terms appeared with greater-than-expected frequency in the Teenage Health Freak corpus (see above). Several text-analysis programs, like WordSmith and AntConc, allow the comparison of a relatively small corpus with a relatively large one, and thus to come to a measure of 'keyness'.

For the sake of simple illustration, let us say that we want to compare the 'carers' corpus' with a larger set of more general spoken conversations and interviews. For this purpose, 10 longer plain-text files have been downloaded from the SCOTS corpus, mainly conversations and interviews with people on topics such as their schooldays, leisure pursuits, academic life, reading habits, weddings and family. The SCOTS corpus contains, at the time of writing, over 1 million words of spoken discourse, of different kinds, ranging from standard English to broad Scots.[4] All the transcripts can be downloaded in plain text format. The sub-corpus of 10 files consists of almost 103,000 words, again a relatively small corpus, but substantial enough to afford a point of comparison with the medical corpus. As in any set of general conversations, it is likely that medical topics might be raised as part of a general corpus, and indeed in Document 805 of the SCOTS corpus, the two participants do begin by talking about their health. The spellings of some items ('oor', 'aboot' represents the speakers' distinctive Scottish accents):

**M816:**    I don't think I ever had rubella, but in our //day it was called German,//

**M815:**    //[laugh] Rubella?//

**M816:**    in oor day it was called German measles, so //ye ye never//

**M815:**    //Ah,// //it's a bit too,//

**M816:**    //bothered aboot it.//

**M815:**    bit too exotic, rubella, don't know, measles.

**M816:**    Mmhm

**M815:**    It's alright.

**M816:**    Aye.

**M815:**    I've never really had a breakage either. I cracked my head open when I was when I was young.

**M816:**    Oh God, I've broken about every bone in my body.'

**M815:**    No.

**M816:**    None o the big, //none o the,//

**M815:**    //Too careful!//

**M816:**    none o the major ones.

Here the two male speakers happen to be sharing memories of illness and accidents; however, most of the conversations are about other topics. What key word analysis promises to reveal, then, are which words in our 'carers' corpus' are unusually frequently used, compared to a corpus of more general conversation that is around 50 times larger. To accomplish this, the 'carers' corpus' and the 10 text-files from SCOTS are loaded into AntConc, which uses a statistical test called 'log-likelihood' to determine which words in the 'carers' corpus' occur unusually frequently. Note that the frequently used words in the lists in the earlier tables are likely to be redistributed in the rankings, since we might expect them to be fairly frequent in both corpora (and so unusually frequent in neither). A high log-likelihood score is given to those items that are 'key' in the 'carers' corpus.' Figure 4.5 shows a screenshot of

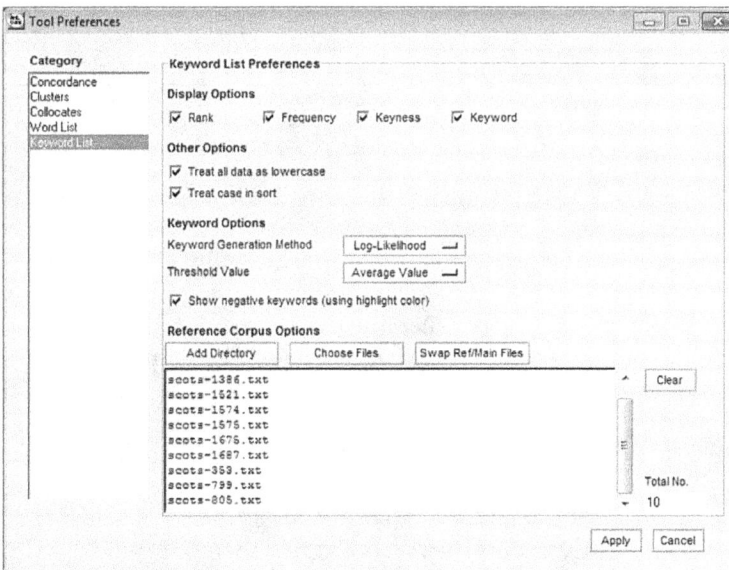

**Figure 4.5** Loading the SCOTS conversations into AntConc

**Table 4.6** Result of keyword analysis of 'carers' corpus' using SCOTS documents as a reference corpus

| Rank | Frequency | Keyness | Keyword |
|------|-----------|---------|---------|
| 1 | 138 | 913.158 | I |
| 2 | 32 | 211.747 | and |
| 3 | 18 | 92.563 | mental |
| 4 | 18 | 87.607 | health |
| 5 | 11 | 72.788 | but |
| 6 | 10 | 66.171 | carer |
| 7 | 11 | 65.978 | cultures |
| 8 | 43 | 63.880 | people |
| 9 | 9 | 59.554 | you |
| 10 | 9 | 53.127 | patient |
| 11 | 9 | 53.127 | treatment |
| 12 | 8 | 52.937 | Amar |
| 13 | 35 | 48.945 | are |
| 14 | 19 | 48.810 | family |
| 15 | 16 | 47.899 | life |
| 16 | 8 | 46.732 | access |
| 17 | 7 | 46.320 | the |
| 18 | 9 | 43.804 | police |
| 19 | 7 | 40.366 | natural |
| 20 | 7 | 40.366 | parent |

AntConc, as the SCOTS documents are being loaded, and Table 4.6 lists the key words in the carers' corpus with respect to the SCOTS conversations.

The results of the keyword search are shown in Table 4.6. The pronouns 'I' and 'you' are still high in the rankings, suggesting that even with respect to conversation more generally, the perspective of speaker and listener are foregrounded in our 'carers' corpus'. The definite article 'the', while frequently used, slips down the rankings to 20th, and many more lexical items come to the fore. These suggest the topics that the seven carers return to again and again, either intensively in a single transcript, or across several transcripts.

The most salient item in the 'carers' corpus' is the highly-frequent term 'I' which apparently occurs even more times than you would normally expect in general conversation. Presumably in interview situations, participants are invited to give personal opinions and 'I' is naturally foregrounded.

Not surprisingly, 'mental' and 'health' occur frequently in the 'carers' corpus', the former in four of the seven interviews, the latter in five. The carers, perhaps because they are from different ethnic backgrounds, have 'cultures' explicitly as a salient issue in the interviews, and, of course, 'carer' and 'patient' rank high in the list of keywords, alongside 'treatment'.

Among the less predictable items in the 'top 20' and the ones that keyword analysis reveals most helpfully to the analyst, are 'family', ranked itself as 14 but semantically grouped with 'parent' at 20. These are carers primarily of family members, but several of the transcripts do focus on different cultural expectations about where the main responsibility for caring lies: whether with the medical authorities or the family. This issue can obviously be a topic for classroom discussion.

Possibly the two most surprising keywords in the analysis, at first glance, are 'police' and 'access.' These results prompt us to return to the texts themselves and combine qualitative analysis of the data with quantitative analysis. A first step to doing this is to use AntConc to do a 'concordance plot', search for each of these items (Figure 4.6). This kind of search, sometimes called a 'dispersion plot' shows where a term occurs in the data, and how it is dispersed within a text.

The concordance plots show that 'police' occurs in only one interview, that of Guo, but that it occurs intensively enough in that interview to identify it as a salient topic in the corpus as a whole. The teacher can then return to and reconsider the data, in which one carer is comparing institutional responses to mental health issues in the United States and the United Kingdom, and suggesting that police officers in the UK be trained to identify mental health patients and that procedures be tightened so that police liaise more closely with members of the community and with medical institutions:

In America, where I come from, you can go to a **police** station and say to the **police**, sir, I have a son who has a mental problem, his name is so and so, his address is so and so. And in case you see him in the stall, or something like that, he needs medical treatment. And the **police** would take down everything. The minute something happen, poom, the **police** will get the ambulance, right into the hospital instead of jail. But you don't have that kind of system here. And the only, – another thing, the policemen are not trained to do all these things. Like my son, the policeman came, he was so rough on him, you know although he has mental problem. The **police** are not trained. The **police** don't know what is mental health. The **police** does not know how sick he is. But, to me, if you, if every community would work with the law enforcement, hand in

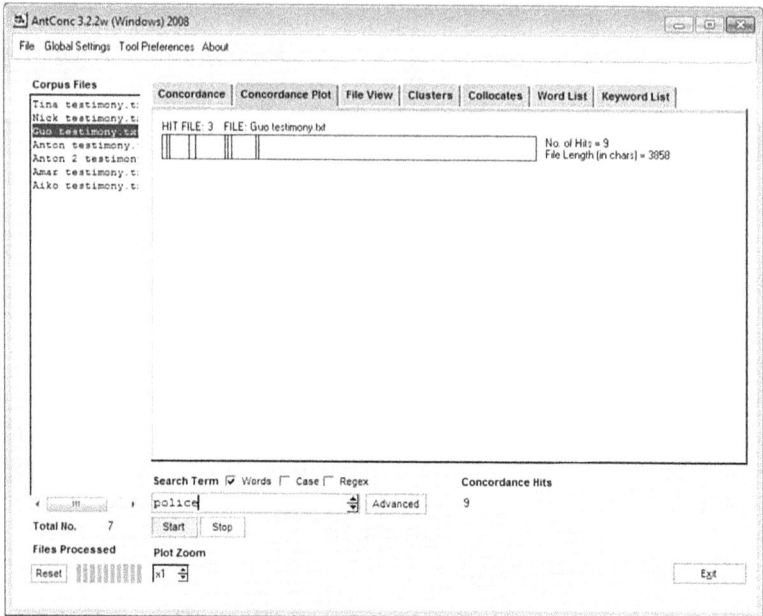

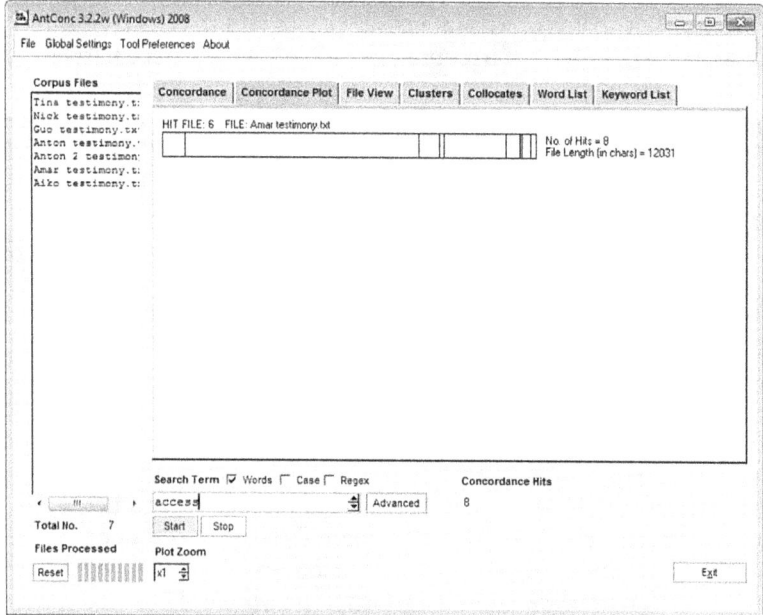

**Figure 4.6** Concordance plots of 'police' and 'access' in the 'carers' corpus'

hand, things might get better, you know. American, some towns, not all, some towns, to me, they are very, very good. I can go the **police** station, and say to **police**, see my son, he's mentally sick. And any trouble, send him to the hospital right away. But then again, here, you can't, you can't send them to hospital. You have to get your doctor. You've got to get psychiatrist. You've got the two policemen. You have to get nurses. You get all, six or seven people have to come before this thing. In America, – poom [claps hands], you go. They save a lot of trouble, you, - they will help the patient too.

This kind of issue, which is clearly of concern to the carer, is a useful one to bring into the medical communication classroom as a scenario for discussion. It raises issues about how various agencies in the community – legal and political – might be integrated; and how the rights and agency of individuals, whether patients or carers, might be affected, beneficially or adversely.

As we have seen, then the term 'police' occurred frequently enough in Gao's interview to become salient in the interview data as a whole. Similarly, the term 'access' occurs intensively – eight times - throughout only one of the interviews, that with Amar. In this case it is interesting to see how she uses the term 'access':

(1)     They say one in four now, it might be more, it certainly feels it more, but awareness and education, easier **access**, people from different communities and different languages, also checking people are doing these things.

(2)     When we are strong we can **access** information, some more easily than others, but we don't always have the strength to listen and look after ourselves and, you know, sooner or later – and it's happening already in health, people are getting conditions they were getting older and now they're getting younger, I mean ...

(3)     Mental health is the same. Children are getting mental health now more and more, we, here in this centre, we see children with all sorts of issues really and mental health is happening earlier and earlier, if ...you weren't born with it, but it's quite easy that anybody can get it and yes, there are some resources and services, but very limited, long waiting lists, not easy to **access**.

(4)     So there needs to be ... Here, at the moment, speaking as a carer and there needs to be more to support, whether it's information or **access**, or talking to somebody, mainly, yes, information and talking to somebody. Information is good help, but talking is even more important, someone to sit and listen, or help you see things clearly,

make you feel worthwhile and maybe assist you to, 'well what about this?'

(5)      Amar thinks statutory services need to be easier to **access** in a crisis.

(6–8)   There needs to be easy **access**, simpler, you know, more resources that people can **access** it when they do need it, not months and years later and also more awareness on whatever illness somebody's trying to look after in a more simpler format, what it is and what they could do. But it's all easily said, but when you're in it, although I know how to **access** more, I have the knowledge, I've experience looking after mentally ill people in my role, it's never easy when it's your own, because you have that power dynamics and attachment.

To sum up, so far, keyword analysis identified 'access' as a salient topic in the sample set of interviews; concordance or dispersion plots revealed that it was intensively used by a single interviewee. Close analysis of the instances of use by that interviewee shows that 'access' means different, albeit related, things to that interviewee: access to information and education about mental health; access to resources and services; access to support within the community. For 'Amar', who is a carer in the community as well as a carer in the family, the concept of 'access' is a crucial factor in her ability effectively to support those for whom she is responsible.

Keyword analysis, then, has the potential to highlight salient topics in texts, spoken or written. Often, keyword analysis will appear to state the obvious, for example that in interview transcripts with carers for patients with mental health challenges the words 'mental' and 'health' will be important. But keyword analysis might also pinpoint topics that are less obvious (except perhaps with hindsight) and thus offers the teacher and learner insights into the concerns of those who produce and consume the texts analysed. Once identified, the terms can be further interrogated, for example using concordance or dispersion plots and close, qualitative analysis of their use in context.

The preceding sections in this chapter have demonstrated different ways of using digital resources to raise teachers' and students' awareness of a key issue in intercultural language education in medical settings: how do professionals and non-professionals use medical language? Frequency analysis, collocation analysis, and the analysis of keywords can show divergent distributions and 'cultural hotspots' in the use of particular terms by groups and individuals. Training in the analysis of digital resources, then, is one potentially exciting way of familiarising students with technical and non-technical terms used in medicine, and raising discussions about appropriate modes of communication.

# Language, Medicine and the Web

The rise of vast quantities of easily-accessible health information on the web, in digital form, has radically changed the relationship between health-care providers and patients. Of course, far from all of the information available on the internet is reliable or trustworthy (cf. Thurlow *et al.*, 2004); even so, there has been a marked trend towards patients presenting at clinics, armed with information about their condition garnered from electronic resources of some kind. By 2005 it was estimated that 117 million Americans, often affluent and often female, were surfing the web for health information before seeing a physician, and they were labelled, somewhat disparagingly as 'cyberchondriacs' (Krane, 2005: 231). In an online article advising practitioners on how to deal with 'web savvy' patients, Anthony (2009) reaffirms the 'low-tech' virtues of personal contact, attention to the parent's anxieties and beliefs, and the face-to-face construction of a planned course of treatment:

> The rise of the Internet has exponentially increased patients' access to health information, potentially altering the patient-physician relationship by raising the level of patients' medical knowledge (and perhaps their level of misunderstanding). While the Internet is a high-tech tool, the key to communicating with web-savvy patients is remarkably low-tech. A patient-centered approach emphasizes understanding patients' concerns, beliefs, and goals, as well as establishing common ground in the development of a mutually understood plan. [http://virtualmentor. ama-assn.org/2009/03/ccas1-0903.html]

Language teachers who work in medical education can also learn from Anthony's advice, and combine the benefits of access to a wealth of digitised discourse on medical and health matters with pedagogical procedures that privilege task-based activities that focus on linguistic and cultural issues. Certainly, materials and course designers, classroom teachers and even learners can develop the technological skills necessary to process and analyse their own digital corpora of medical discourse, interrogating the texts to find common and/or technical expressions for medical concepts, and using a range of techniques to identify recurring or particularly intense cultural concerns that the digitised texts contain. Equally, materials and course designers and classroom teachers can pay attention to research done by others on more specialised corpora of medical language, such as the Teenage Health Freak resource, and note how they provide evidence for the ways in which certain categories of patient articulate both their ailments and (crucially) the world-view and attitudes that shape their perceptions. However, the digital resources themselves are no substitute for the sensitive teacher who recognises the strengths and limitations of the resources, and finds new and imaginative ways of using them to promote language learning and cultural awareness. One important arena for language use that deserves special attention remains face-to-face interaction, and it is to this that we turn in the next chapter.

## Notes

(1)  Medical websites do change their content and, sometimes, addresses. The ones listed here were accessed in early–mid 2011. The addresses are www.aarogya.com (Aarogya in India), www.healthlinks.net (USA), http://www.healthcare.gov (USA), http://www.healthinsite.gov.au (Australia) and http://www.nhsdirect.nhs.uk/ (UK). Wikipedia needs no introduction as an often valuable source of general information that nevertheless sometimes requires its own 'health warning': see http://en.wikipedia.org/wiki/Portal:Health_and_fitness Various websites are designed for patients in general or particular groups: more general sites are http://www.patientvoices.co.uk and http://www.healthtalkonline.org while an age-specific one is the 'Teenage Healthfreak' website at http://www.teenagehealthfreak.org.
(2)  The BYU corpora are freely available at http://corpus.byu.edu; note, however, that users are required to register after a small number of searches.
(3)  The interviews and conversations used in this section are derived from http://www.healthtalkonline.org/mental_health/mentalhealthcarers/People/Stories, and http://www.scottishcorpora.co.uk, while the freely available software, AntConc, designed by Lawrence Anthony, is available to download from http://www.antlab.sci.waseda.ac.jp/software.html.
(4)  Freely available online at www.scottishcorpus.ac.uk The Advanced Search option allows users to download documents in batches.

# 5   Medical Talk

This chapter covers the characteristics and issues arising from different kinds of face-to-face interaction in the broad domain of medicine. Face-to-face interaction between clinicians, nurses and patients, with the possible addition of care-givers and translators, have proved a rich field of research for medical educators, sociologists, linguists and ethnologists, so the present chapter has something of the character of a selective survey of a complex field. The situations and issues we focus on here are:

- Professional–patient communication, particularly in multicultural contexts.
- The use of translators in healthcare communication.
- Professional communication, particularly in the reporting of case histories.
- Non-professional communication, when patients talk about illness.
- Framing spoken discourse in medical communication.
- The issues arising when professionals have to navigate between technical and everyday language, as in interviews for membership of professional associations.

In each of these situations, the participants in the interaction navigate between, across and among cultural boundaries. In professional–patient communication, cultural distance between participants may be the result of difference in geographical, linguistic, class, ethnic or racial background, or difference in age or gender. For example, a younger, Asian male nurse from a middle-class background might be treating an older, female patient who is White and working class in her affiliations and assumptions. They may share English as a *lingua franca*, or they might use a translator as a mediator. If they use a translator, another set of cultural configurations comes into play and contributes to the dynamic of the interaction. Much of the literature on cultural competences in healthcare is about neutralising the potentially harmful effects of communication misfires or prejudicial assumptions based on acknowledged or unacknowledged cultural difference (see Chapter 2). An intercultural approach to healthcare communication assumes that misfires and prejudicial assumptions will necessarily arise out of interaction across cultures. However, the reflective intercultural speaker is trained to be aware of how interaction unfolds, is sensitive to the possibilities of culturally-based misfires and prejudices, and is prepared to use this knowledge to act and adapt where necessary.

Healthcare professionals also need to pay attention to how medical issues are discussed in lay and professional communities: for example, how do particular social and cultural groups talk about healthcare, and how do in-groups of professionals discuss themselves, their work and their patients? The discursive demands on healthcare professionals are many, as they move in and between cultural groups, each with their own presupposed ways of doing things and talking about them. These demands are intensified when the healthcare professional is not a native speaker of English but is required to perform his or her duties in Anglophone contexts. Equally, patients who have to deal with healthcare professionals in what may be their second, third or fourth language need to adopt strategies to present their concerns adequately to those professionals. For the professionals, the demands of moving between the domains of everyday and professional medical discourse are thrown into relief when they have to negotiate unfamiliar and complex situations, such as oral interviews for membership of professional bodies.

To explore the issues arising out of these different situations – professional–patient communication, with or without a translator, doctor talk, patient talk and professional oral examination – we draw here on the substantial research in this area to consider some key concepts in discourse studies:

- the nature of conversational interaction;
- the active role of the translator as mediator;
- means of self-presentation by doctors and patients;
- in-group categorisations;
- medical talk as ideology;
- the importance of framing.

The chapter concludes with some practical suggestions to consider when constructing learning materials that address medical communication across cultures.

# Professional–Patient Interaction as Conversation

In studies of medical communication, conversation analysis (CA) has been a powerful and productive research instrument. Over the past 50 years, coinciding with the increasingly wide availability of recording technologies, CA has developed as a method of exploring the ordered nature of everyday spoken interactions. CA also highlights the ways in which face-to-face interaction articulates participants' interests, motivations and intentions. An article of faith among conversation analysts is that the description of participants' interests, motivations and intentions should be elicited from the fine-grained account of the interaction: the order and management of the participants' 'turns', the length of pauses, the function of non-verbal phenomena like laughter or gasps, and so on. One of the first students of CA, Garfinkel (1967: 1), stresses that data must be 'accountable', that is, the interactions must be closely observed, described and reported in terms that make sense to the participants. Li Wei (2002: 163) sums up the basic tenets of CA thus:

> (i) Social order resides within everyday social life, of which face-to-face interaction is a critical part; (ii) to "know" what people are doing in their everyday life does not require any recourse to hidden motives or models of rationality, but only showing how people actually do it; it then follows that (iii) every claim we as analysts make about what people do must be proven by evidence from the everyday social life of people, which entails a focused, systematic analysis of their face-to-face interaction.

A principle of CA is that external systems of classification should not be imposed onto the interactions. That said, the burgeoning literature on CA has provided analysts with sets of potential frameworks that can help explain how conversation in particular contexts might work. For example, Li Wei (1994, 2002) focuses on the ways in which code switching among Cantonese-English bilinguals functions to accomplish certain conversational tasks. One example (Li Wei, 1994: 163, 2002: 172) shows a mother (A) interacting with her 12-year-old son (B), who is playing with the computer:

**A:**   Finished homework?
**B:**   (2.0)
**A:**   Steven, *yiu mo wan sue?*
      want NEG. PERF. review book
      'Do you want to do your homework?'
**B:**   (1.5) I've finished.[1]

Although it is a brief exchange, this interaction illustrates a number of features of everyday conversation. The mother asks a question, which in context might be taken not as a request for information but as an indirect command: 'Finish your homework'. Questions and commands are among the types of utterance that can have two possible responses, 'preferred' (e.g. the question is answered or the command is accepted), or 'dispreferred' (e.g. the question is not answered or the command is rejected). In CA, many exchanges fall into conventional two-part structures, with a 'preferred' second part (e.g. greeting–greeting, question–answer, request–accept, command–accept) or, alternatively, a 'dispreferred' second part (e.g. the greeting or question might not be acknowledged, or the request or command may be rejected). Here the son's 2.0-second silence is a 'dispreferred' response, provoking the mother to address him directly 'Steven' and reiterate her question/command in Cantonese, here glossed literally and also paraphrased. Again the son produces a dispreferred response: he pauses again, before answering in English, to the effect that he does not need to do his homework. The son's choice of language, contrasting with his mother's, reinforces his non-acquiescence. The interaction, brief though it is, illustrates several features of face-to-face communication that have clear relevance to medical communication, for example, commands in the guise of questions, the management of preferred and dispreferred responses to utterances, the strategic use of silence, and – in intercultural contexts – the loaded value of language choices.

In medical settings, CA has been used extensively in the analysis of healthcare encounters (e.g. Sarangi & Roberts, 1999; Brown et al., 2006: 89–96). Jones (2003, 2009) illustrates its use in nurse–patient communication, and again his analyses show some of the features seen in the mother–son interaction. The interactions between a nurse (**sn**) and a patient (**x**) take the form of a series of questions and answers. Usually, in this case, the questions are not an indirect means of requesting or commanding, but a direct means of eliciting information. Preferred responses give that information in a swift, unproblematical manner; however, there are some non-answers or unexpected answers that count as dispreferred responses. Jones (2003: 614) gives the following illustrative exchange. In the following transcription, short pauses are shown as (.) while longer pauses are shown as numbers of seconds in brackets, e.g. (3.2), the colons (::) indicate a sounds is stretched out, and the words shown between the symbols °...° are spoken more quietly than the words around them:

**sn:**   How-how long do you sleep (.) for?
       (3.2)

**x:**    °Uh:: I wake quite early uhm:: °
**sn:**   How many hours do you sleep at night?
**x:**    Well I try and get 8 hours but its not-its
          not always 11 o'clock umh
          (0.6)
**sn:**   Broken sleep is it
**x:**    I sleep til seven probably yeh yeh
          (0.5)
**sn:**   How many hours a night rough::ly?
**x:**    (.) Say seven um I think
          (7.8) [*sn writes in notes—sleeps seven
          hours a night*]

Like the mother–son interaction, this exchange shows dispreferred responses. The nurse's first question, in this extract, is met by a pause, and a hesitation marker (Uh), both indicators of a dispreferred response. When it comes, the patient's response is quieter than normal, and does not actually answer the question. This prompts the nurse to rephrase the question in more specific terms. Again the patient's response is elusive, more about aspiration than actuality. In his analysis of this sequence, Jones (2003: 615) observes:

Potter (1996) discusses that certain dispreferred turns tend to produce accounts that invoke privileged knowledge. In this case the patient invokes privileged knowledge as to why it might not be possible to answer the question with an exact quantity of sleep. What is noteworthy is that the patient offers the quantity of 8 h as his expectation for a night's sleep, before stating that the time of going to bed is not constant, making it impossible to identify an exact period of time as requested by the nurse. This appears to be the root of the trouble; it is not that the patient does not understand the question, it is that the question does not allow for possible variances of sleep duration.

As the comparison between analyses shows, there are some general similarities in the procedures used to analyse face-to-face conversations in everyday and medical settings. In both the everyday and the medical contexts, analysts pay attention to issues shown in the activity box below.

## Activity: Practising conversation analysis

Ask your students to role play a brief doctor–patient or nurse–patient interview, and record the interaction. Ask the students to transcribe the interaction and then consider the following issues:

(a) Who initiates the sequence and how? What kind of role does the initial turn cast the participants in? For example, in the mother–son exchange, the mother initiates the sequence with a command phrased as a question; in the nurse–patient exchange, the nurse initiates with a question. These opening turns cast the son in the position of accepting or rejecting the command, and the patient in the role of answering or ignoring the question.
(b) How do turns shape the unfolding structure of the exchange? Often the turns fall into conventional pairings such as command–accept, or question–answer.
(c) Are the responses 'preferred' or 'dispreferred'? Preferred responses are characterised by speed of reply, brevity and clarity; dispreferred responses by pausing, hesitation-markers, circumlocution and ambiguity.

Sensitivity to the way interactions unfold and the nuances of conversation are a hallmark of the intercultural speaker. As Li Wei demonstrates, a consideration of the ways in which the mother and son code switch between Cantonese and English is an index of their negotiation of parental authority versus the child's freedom to do as he wishes. And, as Jones shows, the nurse's attention to the patient's dispreferred response might indicate that her question is not one that is easily answered, and that there might be an issue about the regularity of the patient's sleep patterns. However, there are again crucial differences between interactions in everyday and medical settings. The institutional nature of medical communication means that there are ethical and legal considerations that shape the interaction between healthcare provider and patient.

Courses in medical communication, and guides such as Kwong *et al.* (2009) recommend conventional 'scripts' that professionals can use when taking case histories, giving advice, or explaining diseases, drugs, devices, procedures and operations to patients. The 'scripts' are intended to support medical students in assessments such as the Objective Structured (or Standardised) Clinical Examination (OSCE; see www.oscehome.com), part of which takes the form of scenarios in which actors play the role of a patient presenting with some form of disease. The medical student is assessed on how well they deal with the patient. A sample scenario (Kwong *et al.*, 2009: 230) is as follows:

**Doctor role**
You are a foundation year-two (F2) doctor on your surgical rotation. You have been asked to obtain consent, provisionally, from a middle-aged lady who has come in for a laparoscopic cholecystectomy. Your consultant will shortly be up to review what you have told her, but he wants you to start first. You find that her English is not very good.

**Patient role**
You are a middle-aged lady, who has been getting attacks of upper abdominal pain for the past year since coming to the UK from India. When you were admitted 6 months ago, an ultrasound revealed you had gallstones. About 2 months ago the consultant discussed the benefits of an operation to remove the gallbladder, but because it was so long ago you don't remember what he said. You are worried about the operation, since an operation 25 years ago to remove your appendix resulted in a week's stay in hospital, with you needing antibiotics.

Medical students addressing this scenario are advised to obtain consent for the procedure, and check that it is informed, for example, by asking the patient to repeat details of the treatment. The student is also required to explain the benefits and risks 'appropriately'. Again some guidance on phrasing an explanation of laporoscopic cholecycstectomy is given (Kwong *et al.*, 2009: 216–7). The explanation begins:

*We would like to perform keyhole surgery to remove your gall bladder. Previously you had attacks of colicky abdominal pain, caused by your gallstones. We believe that removing the gall bladder will put an end to your symptoms.*

It is obviously a further challenge to explain complex information to patients who do not share the same first language as the healthcare professional. In such instances, Kwong *et al.* (2009: 43–4) suggest 'learning a few basic phrases' of languages commonly used in the community, having a translation sheet ready detailing some common ailments and conditions, assuming the patients are literate in their first language, and using approved advocates and translators (see further, below). However, Skelton (2008: 57) suggests that the 'script' and 'checklist' approach to teaching and assessing communicative skills – an approach that the OSCE tests illustrate – is ill considered, superficial and counterproductive:

> [...] the true function of the checklist is actually to reassure the reader, and beyond the individual reader the discourse community, by offering a clarity and objectivity that are entirely spurious. And, to be clear about this, where such instruments offer advice, we should be aware that such exhortations as 'Maintain appropriate eye contact with the patient' mean 'Look at the patient neither too much nor too little.' This is a game which is not worth the candle.

If the 'checklists' are to have any educational value, they are as prompts to instructors about issues that learners can explore in actual contexts; for example, how much eye contact *is* too much or too little in a given setting between particular interlocutors, who might be discussing a more or less embarrassing condition? Given that CA has shown us the wealth of information that the nuances of conversational exchanges may express, any 'script and checklist' advice that is offered needs to be supplemented by more extensive training in communication. To give overseas doctors support in dealing with healthcare communication in the multicultural setting of Lambeth in London, Moss and Roberts (2003) and Roberts *et al.* (2008) produced two DVDs with accompanying notes on exchanges between doctors and patients from a wide variety of cultural backgrounds. They advocate attention to conversational patterns as a means of sensitising medical students to the strategies required to accomplish effective history taking and explanation. In the following example, a GP (**D**) talks to a Portuguese patient (**P**) who has been hurt at work, when a fire door slammed shut on her ankle:

P:   yes er accident yesterday
D:   ah what was accident
P:   yeah no er
D:   what happened what happened
P:   accident at hotel yesterday
D:   ah you work in the hotel
P:   yes
D:   what is your job Clara
P:   erm yesterday at four o'clock yeah and alarm alarm the uh the er fire
P:   the doors
D:   ah
P:   and er close
D:   right

P:   and in there oof
D:   which er
P:   in the telephone in the sixth floor
D:   right do you work in the hotel
P:   today no
D:   yesterday
P:   yeah
D:   which hotel
P:   er dolphin square hotel
D:   dolphin
P:   square
D:   ah dolphin square hotel
P:   yeah
D:   so: this happened while you were working while you were working
P:   huh oh today no
D:   no yesterday when you were working
P:   erm yeah
D:   what's your job what do you do
P:   erm nine o'clock
D:   no what is your job what is your job
P:   oh job erm
D:   cleaner or
P:   cleaner yeah and er clean the chambermaid
D:   ah chambermaid
P:   yeah sorry
D:   no problem no problem
P:   I understand but er
D:   poco poco eh

As Moss and Roberts (2003: 24) observe, 'Here the doctor and patient have different agendas, which cause them to start "talking past" one another; the GP focuses on the patient's job while the patient wants to talk about her accident'. In CA terms, this means that the exchange is full of 'dispreferred' turns in which the patient either ignores the doctor's question or rejects his conclusion:

D:   what is your job Clara
P:   erm yesterday at four o'clock yeah and alarm alarm the uh the er fire

and

**D:** so: this happened while you were working while you were
working
**P:** huh oh today <u>no</u>

The patient's limited understanding of the English tense system also partially accounts for confusion in time reference (**D**: 'do you work in the
hotel'; **P**: 'today <u>no</u>'). As Moss and Roberts also note, one way in which the
GP does begin to make progress, at least with his own agenda, is by moving
from the kind of open questions consultants are often advised to use ('what
was accident'; 'what happened') to closed questions, either yes/no questions
or either/or questions ('right do you work in the hotel'; 'cleaner or'). These
closed questions focus the conversation by constraining the patient's
possible answers; however, they do not allow her to pursue her own conversational agenda.

The GP's use of a common Portuguese, or, possibly, Spanish phrase
('poco' = *pouco* 'a little') shows him adopting the strategy suggested by
Kwong *et al.* of using common phrases in the patient's own language; however, the educational material that Roberts *et al.* produce is not designed to
provide an all purpose 'script' that healthcare professionals can use in any
consultation. Rather, the DVD materials are designed to show how intercultural communication is embedded in and shaped by contexts that are difficult to predict. Moss and Roberts (2005) further discuss the issues arising
from consultations with patients with limited English proficiency, and they
advocate that general practitioners allow such patients the necessary time to
initiate and develop their own topics, rather than interrupting them in order
to address their own agendas. Allowing patients with limited understanding
of English to direct interaction is not always easy but it has its rewards (Moss
& Roberts, 2005: 417):

> Allowing patients to continue talking when they seem to be straying
> from the intended focus may feel counterintuitive, and challenges GPs'
> strict time constraints. Yet permitting patients to control the topic [...]
> has clear benefits.

Even when patients are given time to control conversational agendas, some
misfires and misunderstandings are inevitable, and so healthcare professionals need to be exposed to intercultural exchanges that are both successful and
unsuccessful. CA can help healthcare professionals reflect on exchanges systematically, in order to develop a flexible set of strategies to improve their
intercultural communicative competence.

# Presenting the Self

Conversation analysis can also help professionals consider how they and their patients are presenting themselves in contexts such as medical consultations. CA theorists consider identity to be, at least in part, socially constructed through interactions in which participants 'position' themselves as particular kinds of 'selves' in relation to 'others'. Intercultural communicative competence involves being aware of how participants draw upon available cultural resources – class, gender, ethnicity, race, as well as stereotypical constructions of the 'sick' role – to position themselves in face-to-face interactions. Burbaum *et al.* (2010: 208) sum up 'positioning' thus:

> In a general sense, positioning refers to discursive practices that people use interactionally to present or construct themselves and others as personae. Central to positioning analysis is the concept of identity. Identity is not considered a static and consistent entity; it is rather seen as locally negotiated and situationally embedded. When doing 'identity work', speakers not only present themselves in a certain way but also 'design' themselves and certain relevant aspects of their identity, which in turn carries certain social consequences. Positioning analysis reconstructs on different levels the verbal actions people use in order to position themselves and to indicate to others how they would like to be seen (self-positioning), and it examines the actions they use to ascribe a certain identity to others (other-positioning).

As various researchers have shown (e.g. Heritage & Stivers, 1999; Mangione-Smith *et al.*, 2003), one way in which professionals and patients negotiate their positions during a medical consultation is through the professional's 'online commentary' on what they are doing. The professional conducts an examination, describing and evaluating as they go along, and so expressing medical authority. The patient may acknowledge, agree or challenge some aspects of this commentary, thus taking up a position in alignment with or opposing the professional's judgement. Heritage and Stivers (1999: 1507) report an exchange that illustrates some of these positioning strategies. A clinician who has been treating a patient for a sinus infection sees him to assess his progress. While the patient persistently positions himself in the 'sick role' (see further, Chapter 6), the clinician uses his own position of authority to reposition the patient as someone who is healthier than he believes himself to be:

**Doc:**   How are you feelin' to[day]:.
**Pat:**                            [·hhh]h Better, hh [hhhhhhhh]

**Doc:**                                                    [And your] sinu[s e [s?]
**Pat:**                                                    [·hh [·h] h
          (.)
**Pat:**   (W)ell they're still: they're about the same
          (.)
**Doc:**   'Bout the sa:me? okay. Why don' I have you sit up here for a second,
          (1.1)
**Doc:**   I gave you a lot of medicine over the la:st (0.5) (general) <u>month</u> or so.
          fer yer <u>sin</u>uses.
          (0.4)
**Doc:**   But the <u>hee</u>mobi::d an' the <u>van</u>cena::se an' then the antibi<u>o</u>tic. the
          augmentin.
          ((0.7)/(·hhhhhh))
**Doc:**   A::nd you <u>should</u> be noticin' a pretty big <u>difference</u>.
**Pat:**   Compared to the first visit, ( ) a lot.
          (.)
**Doc:**   O: [kay.]
**Pat:**      [It's s]till  hhhh ((sniff)) >you know< it's not a hundred percent.
          ((patient continues))

As Heritage and Stivers (1999: 1507) observe, the patient here is attending for
a second consultation, following a first in which he was prescribed antibiotics for a sinus infection. The clinician's initial turns inquire after his health,
and particularly his sinuses; the patient acknowledges that he is feeling
better but states that the sinuses are 'about the same'. The clinician echoes
the patient's evaluation so as to indicate his uncertainty about this judgement, and then readies the patient for examination. As he does so, he lists
the medications prescribed to the patient and states the effect they should
have had ('you <u>should</u> be noticin' a pretty big <u>difference</u>'). The patient
acknowledges that he has noticed a big difference but maintains his position
as 'not a hundred percent'. During the examination, the clinician gives a running commentary that supports his own judgement that the patient should
be feeling much better (Heritage & Stivers, 1999: 1508):

**Doc:**   °Well° I don't see any fluid = your ears look goo:d.
          (3.6)
**Doc:**   This one does too:.
          (5.6)
**Doc:**   Let's see if we see any drainage
          (0.9)
**Doc:**   Say ah::,

**Pat:** Ahh,
(0.2)
**Doc:** An' that looks real good, too:.

Heritage and Stivers (1999: 1510–11) indicate three factors that make it difficult for patients to position themselves in opposition to clinicians' authority: (i) clinicians' professional standing affords them the cultural authority necessary to define and evaluate a patient's condition; (ii) the assessments given during the running commentary are neither conclusive nor offered for discussion; they are incremental positions on the way to a final judgement; and (iii) the comments often address parts of the patients' body that they themselves do not have direct access to. They note that while the patient might continue to resist the clinicians' diagnosis, they seldom contradict their evidence.

The negotiation of a patient's state of health is obviously a key part of any medical consultation. The clinician's confirmation or refutation of evidence of a particular condition will impact on the patient's conception of themselves as healthy or ill. The clinician's verdict may challenge the patient's own self-image and therefore be taken as a threat to be resisted. This is particularly problematical if the clinician's explanation of the patient's symptoms relate to a socially stigmatised cause, or to a set of mental or behavioural causes that affect the patients' construction of their personal identity. The negotiation of identity that we find in CA may also be used as the basis of dramatisations (see further, Chapters 7 and 8). A powerful example of doctor–patient interaction can be found in Tony Kushner's play *Angels in America* ([1992, 1993] 2007: 49–50), in a scene in which the patient, a fictionalised representation of the abrasive US Senator, Roy Cohn, challenges his physician, Henry, who has diagnosed him as suffering from AIDS:

**ROY:** This disease...
**HENRY:** Syndrome.
**ROY:** Whatever. It afflicts mostly homosexuals and drug addicts.
**HENRY:** Mostly. Hemophiliacs are also at risk.
**ROY:** Homosexuals and drug addicts. So why are you implying that I...
*(Pause)*
What are you implying, Henry?
**HENRY:** I don't...
**ROY:** I'm not a drug addict.
**HENRY:** Oh, come on, Roy.
**ROY:** What, what, come on Roy what? Do you think I'm a junkie,

Henry, do you see tracks?

**HENRY:** This is absurd.

In Kushner's play, the physician's diagnosis threatens not only the face but also the career and public reputation of the patient, and the patient resists it fiercely. From real case studies, Burbaum *et al.* (2010) consider the particular challenges arising from psychotherapists' assessment of patients presenting with medically unexplained symptoms that were attributed to psychosomatic causes. Such assessments, as Burbaum *et al.* (2010: 208) acknowledge, also serve to challenge a patients' sense of themselves (that is, 'threaten their face'), by suggesting that they recategorise themselves as patients presenting with a particular kind of physical condition whose cause can be traced to their beliefs and emotions, rather than to an organic cause.

Psychosomatic attributions create a link between the patients' biographical incidents and experiences, their emotions or psychosocial stress factors, and their physical ailments. A psychosomatic attribution can be interpreted as an act of 'other-positioning' in the sense that a patient's experiences and emotions are related to an underlying psychosomatic model, and therefore position the patient as (potentially) psychosomatic.

The means of negotiating 'other-positioning' with patients whose face may be threatened by the attribution of physical symptoms to an alternative, psychological causes are difficult to identify with clarity. Burbaum *et al.* (2010: 211) suggest that the physician tailors the discourse to the individual personality and problems of the patient. The options available to the physician include:

- raising the possibility of alternative explanations early in the consultation, for example, 'Have you noticed any relationship between the stomach pain and stressful meetings that you say you've been having at work?';
- phrasing the alternative attribution in careful, modalised language at a later point in the consultation (e.g. 'Have you considered that your symptoms might possibly come from things that are outside the body?').

While acknowledging that the skilled physician will shape the discursive options to the needs of the patient, Burbaum *et al.* suggest that generally the former strategy might be more patient-centred. That is, explicitly positioning the patient as potentially 'other' at the outset of a consultation, and eliciting a response, can be more productive than the carefully modalised implication later in the consultation. Whichever option is preferred, the competent clinician will realise that offering an explanation of symptoms involves more than the simple exchange of useful information: if the explanation impinges on the patients' sense of self, then the explanation and the recommendations might well be resisted. The interculturally competent clinician, therefore, will be sensitive to this possibility and shape their discourse in the consultation accordingly.

## Mediation in Healthcare Consultations

Face-to-face medical consultations, of course, often involve more people than clinician, nurse and patients. Various potential mediators – caregivers or translators, both informal and professional – can turn the clinician-patient dyad into a triad, with an intricate set of potential consequences that are well documented in studies of interaction within and without the specific domain of healthcare (e.g. Simmel, 1950; Rosow, 1981; Clair, 1990; Hasselkus, 1992; Barone et al., 1999; Baraldi, 2009). The literature shows that mediators, whether caregivers or translators, can impact upon the interaction in a number of ways:

- They can reduce the possibility that patients will share intimate information, for example about embarrassing symptoms or sexual health.
- They can reduce the opportunities for the patient to contribute directly to the interaction; in extreme cases mediators can exclude the patient.
- 'Coalitions' can form between clinician or patient and the mediator. Baraldi (2009) suggests that in consultations involving patients from minority cultures, official translators most commonly form coalitions with the clinician, thus confirming the norms of the host culture.
- Clinicians tend to treat mediators as being more reliable than patients, particularly when the patient is a child or geriatric patient and the mediator is a parent or caregiver (Barone et al., 1999). While mediators can be a useful source of information, the potential is reduced for the child or elderly patient to give voice directly in the consultation.

An illustration of the problems that can occur in mediated interactions is given by Baraldi (2009: 131, original line numbering). Here, a doctor (**D**) addresses a patient (**P**) via a mediator (**M**):

**109  D:** Quanto pesava prima della gravidanza? (*How much did she weigh before getting pregnant?*)

**110  M:** Before this pregnancy, how many of we – what was your weight?

**111  P:** Eighty.

**112**   **M:** Eighty?
**113**   **D:** Quanto? (*How much?*)
**114**   **M:** No. Before the pregnancy. Before the pregnancy.
**115**   **D:** Prima, prima di diventare grassa (*Before becoming fat*)
**116**   **M:** When you were not pregnant.
**117**   **D:** No.
**118**   **M:** Eighty? Are you sure?
**119**   **D:** No:: ottanta? No:: troppo. (*No, eighty? No, too much*)
**120**   **M:** It can't be. It can't be eighty. No, no. (5)
**121**   **D:** Beh? Quanto pesavi? (*So? How much did you weigh?*)
**122**   **M:** You can't remember.

As Baraldi (2009: 131) observes, the clinician does not question the patient directly, but through the mediator. The mediator translates the question (turn 110) but when the patient replies, the mediator questions the information (turn 112). The clinician repeats his question, and he and the mediator elaborate upon it and check until, in turn 119, the clinician finally casts doubt on the patient's response. The mediator, in turn 122, interprets the patient's response as an inability to remember the information accurately, although, as Baraldi (2009: 131) informs us, later examination of the medical records confirms that the patient had indeed lost weight during her pregnancy. Here, both clinician and mediator form a coalition, and treat the patient as an unreliable informant. Baraldi (2009: 134) concludes:

> Mediators might become more aware of the importance of their formulations in translation and of their empowerment of patients' active participation. Healthcare providers might: (1) actively and effectively help mediators in their coordination of the interaction, e.g. explicitly asking for more accurate information about patients' needs, worries or doubts; (2) actively co-coordinate the interaction, e.g. encouraging patients' utterances in their second language, and using patients' most recurrent lexicon.

In the light of such behaviour in encounters involving mediators, medical educators are increasingly developing materials to achieve the aspirations expressed above by Baraldi. For example, the California Endowment, a private foundation that supports healthcare for marginalised communities in the state of California, has devised and published manuals and workbooks that raise participants' awareness of issues in healthcare translation and mediation.[2] The manual and workbook give mediators advice and scenarios for practice consultations, based on a set of principles and standards for healthcare translation and mediation. One of the explicit roles identified in the manual and workbook is that of 'cultural clarifier', which can be related to Byram's concept of the intercultural speaker as mediator between languages and cultures. In clarifying miscommunication that can arise out of cultural misalignments, mediators are encouraged to conform to the standards and performance measures suggested by the California Healthcare Interpreters Association (2002: 31–32):

> Interpreters seek to understand how diversity and cultural similarities and differences have a fundamental impact on the healthcare encounter. Interpreters play a critical role in identifying cultural issues and considering how and when to move to a cultural clarifier role. Becoming culturally sensitive and culturally responsive is a life-long process that begins with an introspective look at oneself.

**Performance Measures**

Interpreter demonstrates cultural responsiveness by seeking to:

(a)   Identify and monitor personal biases and assumptions that can influence either positive or negative reactions in him/her, without allowing him/her to impact the interpreting.
(b)   Recognize and identify when personal values and cultural beliefs among all parties are in conflict.
(c)   Monitor and to prevent personal reactions and feelings, such as embarrassment or frustration, that interfere with the accuracy of the message, and to recognize such reactions may be similar to or different from the patient and provider.
(d)   Identify statements made by providers and patients indicating a lack of understanding regarding health beliefs and practices, and to use applicable strategies suggested in the cultural clarifier role to prevent potential miscommunication.
(e)   Seek continually to update their knowledge and understanding of the dynamic cultures of patients, healthcare providers, and the culture of the healthcare system in the United States.

Of course, not all mediators are provided by institutions, trained or supported. Hasselkus (1992: 301–302) focuses on the role of the family caregiver in consultations with geriatric patients, noting that such mediators tend to adopt discursive strategies that conform to the functions of 'Facilitators', 'Intermediaries' or 'Direct Sources' of information.

Much of the data in the 'Facilitator' category represent efforts by the caregiver to translate the medical world to the patient ('Your eyedrops, mother') and the patient's lifeworld to the doctor ('She's talking about the prednisone'). One might call this a monolingual analogy to bilingual translation. In the 'Intermediary' category, the caregiver shifts between serving as a patient substitute and doctor substitute, clearly having one foot in each world and trying to provide a bridge of communication between the two worlds. In 'Direct Source', the juxtaposition of the two worlds within the caregiver is even more pronounced as the caregiver replaced the patient in a dyad with the physician, becoming the solitary voice of the lifeworld, and then attempted to be the voice of medicine as he or she shifted into the practitioner role with the patient. In mediating activities, the caregiver again served as the bridge between the different views represented by the two worlds. And finally, in culture brokering, the caregiver introduced the patient's lifeworld context into the medical interview.

The mediator, then – whether trained or not – plays the key role of 'intercultural broker'. The healthcare professional needs to be aware of the mediator's agency in the triadic encounter, and that the mediator may well arrive at the consultation with a set of preconceptions or, indeed, his or her own agenda. The clinician or nurse, then, needs to take account of the status of the mediator and the various roles he or she might play in the consultation, and to give the patients sufficient space and opportunity to articulate, as best they can, their own concerns directly as full participants in the discourse.

# Doctor–Doctor Talk

Not all medical discourse involves patients or mediators. In various contexts, healthcare professionals discuss patients in groups of their peers. 'Doctor talk' or 'nurse talk' occurs, for example, when junior doctors or nurses are presenting case studies to more experienced colleagues. And, in the following section, we discuss situations in which non-professionals discuss medical topics.

At Kaohsiung Medical University, for example, medical students and junior doctors discuss case studies with senior colleagues. At one such presentation, observed by one of the authors,[3] around 18 doctors were present. Although all of the doctors were Taiwanese, much of the presentation was in English, with a switch to Chinese towards the end of the session. The seating arrangements provided a clue to seniority, with junior doctors clustered at the front, more senior colleagues situated further back. One junior doctor presented a case, which involved a patient with suspected cancer having a tumour removed. The presenter used Power Point slides and others contributed with comments. The case presenter used the language of medicine to describe shapes and sizes, express possibilities, give intentions ('I'm going to...') and ask for suggestions ('Should the patient receive...?'). The others contradicted ('I have another opinion'), requested clarification ('Do you mean...?'; 'That means...?'), asked for justification ('Why?') and expressed scepticism ('I don't think...'). The doctors used laser pointers to refer to salient features on the images displayed on the slides. The most senior physician present played the role of tutor, asking questions and checking facts and procedures ('What's your opinion?'; 'What kind of tests did you carry out?'; 'What are the criteria for the tests?'; 'How do you know...?'). He also provided a summary and evaluation of the presentation. After the presentation, he looked at a list of medical students' names and photographs, and nominated particular students to answer specific questions about the case, throwing open the discussion to others with the cue, 'Any comments?' As well as asking questions about the diagnosis and surgical procedures, there was reflection on the ethics of the case. The patient in question was apparently a heroin abuser: had the junior doctors checked the insurance situation, and how would they proceed if the patient refused a further examination?

Through such interactions, which may well be in the second language, the medical student is socialised into the procedures and also the values of the professional community. Students and junior doctors are required to display their competence through their presentations, challenges and responses; as they move up through the hierarchy, their physical locations and roles in the speech event change.

The contexts in which students and junior doctors are required to display competence may vary from context to context; however, the challenges, and the strategies adopted to address them may be similar across the profession. Research in the United States in the 1980s suggested that native speaker, junior medical staff were also aware that their public face was at stake when they were quizzed by senior colleagues, or 'attendings', when they were doing the rounds of hospital wards (Anspach, 1988: 362):

> You gotta put on an air so that you will convince the attendings that you know about the case, and that you're smarter than they are. You've gotta display an air of confidence. (How do you do that?) You show confidence by the way you talk. (How do you talk?) You don't stop between sentences, you don't hesitate. They don't want to see you flipping through the chart. If you make a mistake in the hemoglobin value, don't say it was a mistake.... If you have to say "I don't know," don't apologize for

it or say it unconfidently. You can say, "I don't know," but it has to be done in the right way, like nobody else would know either, not like you should've known. Just keep up the flow so you don't get interrupted.

Anspach showed that medical students were encouraged to construct a public persona that combines confidence with a degree of appropriate honesty and humility when caught in error. This kind of insight informed understanding of the 'hidden curriculum' of medical education, as it was made manifest:

> not only [in] lectures in the classroom, small group discussions, exercises in the laboratory, and care for patients in clinic but also [in] conversations held in the hallway, jokes told in the cafeteria, and stories exchanged about a 'great case' on our way to the parking lot'. (Stern & Papadakis, 2006: 1794)

Changes in medical education and an increased focus on professional conduct (reinforced by professional codes and charters, such as that published by the Members of the Medical Professionalism Project, 2002) have put a critical spotlight on, say, the kinds of 'gallows humour' reported to be a characteristic of doctors' informal discourse in the 1970s (e.g. Coombs & Goldman, 1973; see also Chapter 7). In the developing discourse on standards of professional conduct in medical education, Stern and Papadakis argue for the necessity for providing explicit and formal opportunities for reflection alongside observation of professional behaviour that may be considered correct or incorrect. Prompts for reflection may include the behaviour of senior physicians who are considered role models, or indeed the language and behaviour of more junior peers. They recommend that physicians' memoirs and 'parables' or 'storytelling' also represent an instructive basis for the discussion of professional behaviour and the internalisation of core values that lead to compassionate communication. As Stern and Papadakis (2006: 1796) note:

> [...] modeling professional behavior on the part of a teacher (e.g. showing compassion to a dying patient or offering reassurance about recovery) without following up with discussion constitutes a missed opportunity for teaching professionalism.

Stern and Papadakis acknowledge that finding occasion to build reflection into a formal curriculum is a challenge. However, at some point in the medical education syllabus, there has to be space for critical reflection that addresses the discourse of formal case presentations and doctor–patient consultations, as well as the informal conversations and jokes related by healthcare practitioners to each other. Chapters 7 and 8 of the present volume offer some suggestions for incorporating storytelling – based on literature and the visual arts – into medical education as means of encouraging reflection on issues of communication and professional values.

## Patient Talk: Everyday Beliefs

Several times in this and the previous chapter we have contrasted the differing attitudes, values and concerns of professionals and non-professionals when communicating about medical topics. Balshem (1991) illustrates a methodology for participant observation of non-professional medical talk within, in her case, a relatively deprived inner city, working class community in the United States. Balshem acted as a health worker in the community and engaged its inhabitants in discussions about the nature and causality of heart disease and cancer. By recording and analysing the discussions, she built up a picture of the mythologies – that is, the everyday beliefs and values – relating to these conditions in the community, and suggested some reasons why the members of the community tended to reject health advice about diet and smoking projected by the medical professionals and institutions. Particularly in the case of cancer, she found a tendency towards fatalism in the community, combined with a perspective that valued personal individualism, stoicism and courage in the face of adversity. These values were dramatised through anecdotes of illness such as the following (Balshem, 1991: 163):

> Like my father – he had leukemia, which is cancer of the blood. They told him that he only had two months to live, and he says, "No way – I'm makin' that summer because I'm going to my boat." And the doctors still can't believe to this day that he made four months.... And he died at the end of September. So I think outlook has a lot to do with it. If you make up your mind you're going to do something about it, you can.... He was a fighter.

This kind of story has features in common with many non-professional narratives of illness. The individual benefits from courage and perseverance against a cruel fate: the individual will triumphs, if temporarily, over the disease. Often, the courage of the individual is shown to invalidate the so-called 'professional wisdom' of the medics, making nonsense of their predictions. 'Outlook', determination, and a goal in life ('I'm going to my boat') are seen as factors that can, again temporarily, diminish the impact of disease. As Balshem (1991: 166) argues, the illness narrative in the non-professionals' culture is often a narrative about authority and control:

> Community residents assert local control of the value ascribed to local tradition. With regard to beliefs about cancer, their assertions are made in the context of powerfully emotional issues surrounding fate, suffering, life, and death. What is being negotiated is authority: the authority to judge local belief and activity concerning cancer, control, and causality.

The portrayal of medicine as conflict between the authority of non-professionals and professionals is not confined to the inner cities of the United States. The activity below is based on a transcript from a longer conversation between a Scottish mother (F634) and her daughter (F631). The mother tells of an incident when she was a younger woman, suffering from encephalitis, an infection that impaired her memory and caused seizures.

---

## Activity: Analysing a medical anecdote

Look at the following excerpt from a conversation between a mother and her daughter [source: www.scottishcorpus.ac.uk: Document 350; Interview 04]. Consider the way the mother portrays herself and her family, and contrast it with the way she describes professional clinicians.

**F634:**   I was taking fits. So they weren't quite sure if the fits would would happen again. So, therefore, you know, I wasn't, it wasn't a good idea to be just in charge of Gillian by myself. So, I stayed at gran's for a couple of weeks and then I started to get really quite well erm and, of course, wanted home. And that was when I started to go on the homeopathic medication erm because papa wasn't happy about the strong drugs I was takin. I was havin to take these strong drugs. and I went on the homeopathic medication. And when I went back to s- for my outpatient appointment at ehm the hospital, saw one [burp] excuse me, one of the surgeons, Mr. Jamieson. He was amazed. He was totally amazed [cough] that I had made such a good recovery, because evidently this encephalitis can, it ah, it can i- it's not likely to end your life, but it can e- end your active life, you know, it could it could

---

interfere with your quality of life. ehm and it didn't interfere with my quality of life after a while, but that was havin got the strong drugs out of my system, only to replace them with homeopathic medication. And now, I I didn't own up to the fact that I was erm not taking the drugs. Cause they just said, 'Are you still taking your medication?' And I just said, 'Yes.' 'Well, you're doing remarkably well,' says the and I reme-, this is one thing I do remember [inhale] eh the room was full of students, you know, obviously medical students, when when he was interviewing me. and he said to one, to the d- to the students, 'Anybody got any questions to ask Mrs Ower?' And this young student said to me ehm, 'Do you manage to read Mrs Ower?' And I said ehm, 'Yes.' He said, 'What do you read?' And I said, 'Well, I read the papers.' And he said, 'Do you?' And I said 'Aye'. He says, 'Tell me what's in the papers just now? What's happening, you know, what's, sort of, in the headlines just now?' And I said ehm, 'Martin Luther King's been assassinated.' So that kind of puts a a date on it, doesn't it?

**F631:** mmhm

**F634:** And he he just looked at me and he said, 'hmm'. So I think they were testing //me,//

**F631:** //mm//

**F634:** you see, to see if I, in fact, did read the papers.

**F631:** mmhm

**F634:** And I did, because I was so sad about that, you know, that was a tragedy,

**F631:** mmhm

**F634:** ehm a a complete tragedy ehm, so I remember that. So I think that gave me a lot of brownie points. And I said to him, 'could I get my t- do, get to drive now? Can I get my licence back?' Cause they they took my my licence, wasn't allowed to drive, and Mr Block, eh Mr Jamieson it was, and he said, 'No, no.' He said, 'I think we'll give you another six months before we're comfortable with the driving.' So I went back in six months and I I was almost fu- fully restored. I think I was fully restored to to, you know, normal health again, erm, and then I got my licence back and he said to me, 'Well, there's nothing we can do

> Mrs Ower. We just need to discharge you.' He said, 'Normally
> people like you are coming back here for years, and years.'
> erm, and he said, 'But, you know, you seem to have made
> such a good recovery.' He said, 'I think you've had youth
> on your side. You know, you're young,
>
> **F631:** mm
> **F634:** and you're normally healthy. So you've picked up this
> infection and, okay it's it's, you know, it's laid you low, but
> your actual recovery period has been very good.' But, I still
> never mentioned the homeopathic medicine. I just kept
> takin it.

As the anecdote is told, the mother's narrative dramatises a conflict between the ignorance of the professionals ('they weren't sure if the fits would happen again') and family wisdom ('papa wasn't happy about the strong drugs I was takin'). The narrator assumes control of her own healthcare by taking homeopathic medication rather than the prescribed drugs, and, as in Balshem's example, we find the recurring trope of medical authorities being 'amazed, totally amazed'. The narrator's courage is implicit in her reliance on homeopathic medicine in the face of a serious illness ('it can end your active life'), but vindication comes in the form of her passing the medical students' test ('I think that gave me a lot of brownie points', that is, marks of approval for having done something good) and being regarded as exceptional by the doctor ('normally people like you are coming back here for years'). The narrator's self worth is boosted by her belief – or privileged knowledge – that it was not her youth but her use of folk medicine that accounted for the speed of her recovery.

What the professional and non-professional peer-group discourses have in common is an ambivalent portrayal of the other 'culture'. Medical professionals can fall into the discursive habit of depersonalising individual patients, and even characterising them as contemptible or worthless: 'gomers' and 'crocks' (see further, Chapter 7). These characterisations co-exist with the unarguable fact that physicians and nurses belong to caring professions. Equally, lay folk depend on doctors and go to them for assistance and self-validation. But they also characterise them as oppressive authorities whose professional qualifications mask a fundamental ignorance and impotence. And, given that lay narratives privilege folk wisdom and strength of individual character over prescribed remedies, it is hardly surprising that an issue in healthcare is non-adherence to courses of treatment negotiated with the physician.

Interculturally competent mediators will be aware of how such discourses work, and the potential that they possess for stereotypical characterisations leading to communicative mismatches. Professionals and lay people belong to different cultures insofar as they organise their experience according to different sets of expectations, or 'frames' (cf. Agar, 1994: 134–135). In Agar's terms, frames can be conceptualised as default expectations, in our case that patients should or should not follow physicians' or parental advice when dealing with serious illness. Intercultural mediators recognise difference and attempt to align frames so that each side can negotiate from a common set of understandings. However, this kind of alignment of frames is not an easy task to accomplish. The next section considers strategies for dealing with mismatched expectations between speakers of different languages who are communicating in medical settings.

# Intercultural Framing

The following exchange (Cameron & Williams, 1997: 427) between a non-native speaker, a Thai nurse working in the United States, and an American Alzheimer's sufferer serves as a simple example of miscommunication arising from mismatched frames. Here the nurse wants to test the word recall of an early-stage Alzheimer's sufferer:

**Nurse:**      OK. And you know what is? *[Pointing to watch on her wrist]*
                What is?
**Patient A:**  Huh? Quarter after ten.
**Nurse:**      Oh. OK. What is?
**Patient A:**  It's a watch.

Here we see the patient switching from the 'everyday' frame to the 'professional' frame. If someone points to his or her wrist and asks a question, the normal response is to give the time. As Cameron and Williams observe, in relevance theory this understanding requires least processing. The switch to a 'professional medical' frame, in which the patient is actually being tested on word recall, requires more processing – but this patient accomplishes the task once it becomes evident to him that the time is not what the nurse requires. Note that the nurse's level of English is an issue here – her question is ill formed with respect to native-speaker norms – but better formed phrasing would not necessarily have resolved the problem. The nurse's level of English proficiency is not, in fact, a serious obstacle to her successful communication in many instances. Because she is usually in the same 'frame' as the patient or doctor, all the conversational participants use their subject knowledge, such as it is, to resolve breakdowns (Cameron & Williams, 1997: 430):

**Nurse:**     We (first start on) that part. I would like to answers some family history from you.
**Patient B:**  OK.
**Nurse:**     Because I would like to know you more and more.
**Patient B:**  OK.
**Nurse:**     mmhm ... uh ... Are you married?
**Patient B:**  Nooo.
**Nurse:**     Uh ... how many [sibrins] do you have?
**Patient B:**  How many children?
**Nurse:**     Sibr – I mean brother and sister.
**Patient:**    Oh siblings. OK. OK. None. Well I ain't got to think about that. I don't have any brothers or sisters. No brothers or sisters.

Here the nurse uses a relatively uncommon word with an unfamiliar pronunciation. The patient uses the 'family history' frame to make an informed guess about meaning, and the nurse realises that miscommunication has occurred. She therefore begins to repeat and then paraphrases her original question. Given the paraphrase, the patient realises the meaning of the original question and answers it.

The importance of establishing a framework for the interpretation of utterances is also evident in research into the oral assessment of overseas doctors. Roberts *et al.* (2000) considered candidates from ethnic minority – largely Asian – communities, who were taking an oral test for membership of the Royal College of General Practitioners (RCGP). Echoing Cameron and Williams, Roberts *et al.* (2000: 371) realised in their research that:

> The language of the oral examinations is not a transparent medium through which information passes, but a set of discourses that actively construct a particular way of looking at the world. The different ways in which clinical practice is talked about, in different institutional and professional domains and by different groups, produces a range of discourses that call up particular types of vocabulary, metaphor and grammatical constructions and certain lines of argument and representation.

Roberts *et al.* analysed the responses and grades given to candidates' answers to questions such as:

•  What does the concept 'patient-centredness' mean to you?
•  What strategies would you use for coping with uncertainty?

• A young chap of 26 who has difficulty with sleeping comes to see you. How does that make you feel?

The interesting thing about these questions is that they can be answered according to several possible 'frames'. In this respect, they are like the simple question 'How are you?' when asked by a doctor to a patient at the start of a consultation: the question can be understood within a personal frame as a polite greeting, or within a professional frame as a request for medical information. Roberts *et al.* (2000: 371) identify three types of 'frame' or discourse that operate – to the candidates' advantage or disadvantage – in the RCGP medical examinations. They are summarised below:

*Personal experience* – talk about the individual's experiences and feelings; characterised by particular examples and the telling of anecdotes, reminiscences, etc.

*Professional discourse* – talk of 'shared ways of knowing and seeing that characterise the community of medical practitioners'; characterised by doctor-doctor discussions and doctor-patient consultations.

*Institutional discourse* – a more abstract level of talk in which GPs account for their values, attitudes and behaviour in examinations, departmental meetings, quality assessments, etc.

The RCGP oral examinations contained all three types of discourse; however, it was the more abstract institutional discourse that was privileged by the assessors and marked most highly. So, for example, a personal response to the following question was discounted by the examiners, whose follow up question demanded a more institutional response (Roberts *et al.*, 2000: 373):

**Examiner:**    A young chap of 26 who has difficulty with sleeping comes to see you. How does that make you feel?

**Candidate:**    It feels like a threatening consultation. It's a difficult consultation. It's quite possible to encounter a difficulty in the beginning. 'I'm sorry you can't sleep. I remember when my child was little.'

**Examiner:**    Can you briefly list alternative ways?

Here the examiner sounds as if he is operating within a 'personal' frame, identifying a particular situation, and requesting information about feelings. The candidate responds within the personal frame, but the examiner's follow up question indicates that he is actually operating in an institutional frame, requesting a list and evaluation of alternative ways of dealing with a young man with insomnia.

Roberts *et al.*'s research into the RCGP assessments suggest that non-native-speaker candidates, like the Thai nurse in her conversations with patients and doctors, do not struggle so much with language forms as with the task of making sense of discourse within the appropriate frame. The importance of contextual knowledge has for some time been apparent in the teaching of listening and comprehension skills; for example, Ridgway (2000: 182) observes that:

> Native speakers only recognize individual words which have been spliced out of a text, approximately half the time, (Lieberman 1963), so word comprehension must be far more dependent on co-text and context in listening than it is in reading. Top-down processes must play a more important part in (fluent) listening than in reading.

In the context of medical examinations, Roberts *et al.* (2000: 373) identify real difficulties for overseas candidates when choosing an institutional frame to deal with the following areas:

• Values and attitudes – where values and attitudes differ from those operating in the UK, overseas candidates can feel at a disadvantage. They may be sensitive to the fact that conventions governing, for example, childbirth, might be different in the UK and their home country.
• Cultural difference – related to the topic of values and attitudes, there are key subjects, such as contraception, abortion and sexual activity, that will vary from community to community. The successful candidate has to be able to disengage from personal discourse and to discuss these issues in a manner appropriate to the institutional frame.
• Acknowledging uncertainty – in an assessment there are areas where the candidate might legitimately not know the resolution to a problem. The challenge in the institutional frame of an assessment is to show that this uncertainty is not to do with the individual's failings but with the general state of the medical profession.

The intercultural language educator has to be aware, then, of the different demands of different genres of general and professional discourse. The intercultural healthcare professional is required to be sensitive to the way individuals interact in different settings, and to the ways in which they relate and interpret information. One characteristic that is key to the success of much professional discourse is the strategic development of *explicitness*. Medical practitioners can promote explicitness in two ways:

- Learners of English can raise their language proficiency to the point where they can skilfully negotiate the meaning in dynamic interaction.
- Both learners at different levels of proficiency *and* native-speakers of English can develop strategies, even when their language proficiency is limited, to provide contextual clues to the kind of frames within their interlocutors will understand their utterances.

We conclude this chapter by offering three examples of how explicitness may be achieved in medical communication. The first example we have already seen. The nurse from Thailand is questioning an elderly American patient about his history. Although her English is not at a high level she is careful to establish the frame of 'family history' clearly, and this frame allows the patient to make informed guesses as to the nurse's meaning even when he does not understand her pronunciation:

**Nurse:**         We (first start on) that part. I would like to answers some family history from you.
**Patient B:**   OK.
**Nurse:**         Because I would like to know you more and more.
**Patient B:**   OK.
[. . .]
**Nurse:**         Uh . . . how many [sibrins] do you have?
**Patient B:**   How many children?

In the second example, also from Cameron and Williams (1997: 426) the Thai nurse and an American preceptor (an experienced registered nurse who is supervising her) are discussing a patient who is suffering from post-traumatic stress disorder. In the terms of Roberts *et al.*, this is a 'professional frame' and both participants are aware of this. Even so, the Thai nurse's pronunciation of a particular word [tam = time or term] causes her preceptor problems:

**Nurse:**          uh recent history he started on amitriptyline HS two [tams]
                         And then he has uh short [tam] therapy
                         one [tam] before he came here
**Preceptor:**   What-what do you mean by short-term therapy, [Name of nurse]?
**Nurse:**          He uh short [tam] therapy.

| | |
|---|---|
| **Preceptor:** | At uh ou-out patient clinic? |
| **Nurse:** | Yea |
| **Preceptor:** | Yea, like how many weeks or days? |
| **Nurse:** | Just one [tam] |
| **Preceptor:** | o-oh one time |
| **Nurse:** | One [tam] by Dr D. |
| **Preceptor:** | mmhhmm. So he saw him once. |
| **Nurse:** | mmhm |
| **Preceptor:** | For two days, before he came? |
| **Nurse:** | umm |
| **Preceptor:** | You said twice. |
| **Nurse:** | Yes, twice. |
| **Preceptor:** | I didn't know what that meant. So he had that for two, just two days of that. |

The issue here is that the nurse's pronunciation of [tam] could be interpreted as *time*, in which case the preceptor should understand that the patient had two doses of the drug on consecutive days, or it could be interpreted as *term*, in which case the preceptor should understand that the patient had two full courses of the drug. And again, does the nurse mean that the patient received therapy for a short *term* (that is, a single visit to a therapist) or a short *time* (perhaps several visits over a limited period)?

There are various ways in which this kind of difficulty could be resolved. The nurse could strive to acquire a rhotic accent which would help disambiguate *time* and *term*. Or the preceptor could ask more explicit questions. Look again at the exchange:

| | |
|---|---|
| **Preceptor:** | What-what do you mean by short-term therapy, [Name of nurse]? |
| **Nurse:** | He uh short [tam] therapy. |

The preceptor's open question is an unusual one for professional discourse – it looks more like the kind of question you would find in an institutional setting such as an examination. The nurse clearly does not know how to answer it, or what the preceptor's problem is, and so she simply repeats herself. The preceptor then asks what language teachers call two 'concept' questions, in an attempt to elicit the location and duration of the therapy:

| | |
|---|---|
| **Preceptor:** | At uh ou-out patient clinic? |
| **Nurse:** | Yea |

**Preceptor:**   Yea, like how many weeks or days?
**Nurse:**   Just one [tam]
**Preceptor:**   o-oh one time

The dialogue as a whole shows the preceptor asking a number of clarification and checking questions to ensure that the meaning is conveyed accurately. Such questions are evidently an important part of making medical communication explicit.

A further strategy to promote explicitness is the avoidance of indirectness when asking questions. Indirectness seems to be a feature of institutional discourse in the UK, particularly in oral assessments, test or interviews, in which an indirect question that *appears* to be personal is generally regarded as a polite means of inviting the candidate to expand on their knowledge and skills within an institutional frame. This shift from personal to institutional does seem to be difficult for many candidates, as we can see from the following example from Roberts *et al.* (2000: 372). The examiner here is forced to move from an apparently personal frame to an explicitly institutional frame, in what Roberts *et al.* call 'an uncomfortable moment' which could have been avoided if the examiner had asked the explicit version of the question ('How do you find out what a patient wants from the service?') in the first place:

**Examiner:**   What do patients feel like when they are ill?
**Candidate:**   [No response]
**Examiner:**   What does illness make you feel? Fear? Pain?
   How do you find out what a patient wants from the service? That's what I'm getting at...

The activity below draws on several of the issues dealt with so far in this chapter: it draws on a simulation, a 'critical incident' in which a patient who is also a nurse requests medication and help from a senior nursing colleague.[4] In this dialogue, they negotiate their professional identities and their responsibilities to each other both as colleagues and patient-nurse.

## Activity: Self-presentation and framing

The dialogue below is extracted from a longer exchange between a patient (who is also a nurse) and a senior nursing colleague. It shows the patient making two difficult requests of her colleague, and the colleague dealing with them in a sympathetic but non-committal way. Read the dialogue and consider the following questions:

(1)  How does the patient frame her request for the painkiller, DF118?
(2)  How does the nurse express her refusal?
(3)  How does the patient then frame her desire to sue the health board?
(4)  How does the nurse offer alternative ways of understanding the patient's problems at work?

**NURSE:**     What can I help you with today? I noticed you were very sore coming in there.
**PATIENT:**   Yeah. I'm having another back episode.
**NURSE:**     Oh are you?
**PATIENT:**   Ehm
**NURSE:**     Right.
**PATIENT:**   it just flares up every now and again when there's something sort of stressful going on.
**NURSE:**     Okay.
**PATIENT:**   Ehm so, getting a lot of work done in the house just now and it seems to just sort of gone ping. I'm off sick again with it.
**NURSE:**     Right, and have you seen the doctor to get painkillers or anything?
**PATIENT:**   He gave me, ehm I did see him, ehm the last time that this happened and he gave me a prescription for DF118 to take on the top of the Neurofen and the Paracetamol.
**NURSE:**     Uh-huh
**PATIENT:**   Ehm
**PATIENT:**   And it takes the edge off it but it's not really, it's
**NURSE:**     Okay.
**PATIENT:**   not going anywhere, do you know what I mean? Ehm, so I need to do something about this, <*name*>. I ca- I can't go on. I mean there's, it gets more and more frequent. The attacks are more close together now and it's just I've had enough.
**NURSE:**     Okay.
**NURSE:**     So you've not, eh, cos you'd asked specifically to come and see me today.
**PATIENT:**   Yeah.

**NURSE:** And I'm obviously very concerned about your back pain but I would pre- for things like giving a prescription, as a nurse practitioner I can't give you something like DF118.

**PATIENT:** Nope.

**NURSE:** Eh, but I'll, I'll certainly get you to see the GP today, once we're finished. But I, I, I,

**PATIENT:** Okay.

**NURSE:** y-you know? I know you'd wanted to see me specifically, was there another reason you wanted to see me today?

**PATIENT:** Yeah because <exhales> I've had enough of the I mean that's, it's eh virtually impossible to do the job properly. I mean you –

**NURSE:** You're still, you're still nursing, aren't you?

**PATIENT:** you know the word that I want. Yeah.

**NURSE:** Yeah.

**PATIENT:** Yup.

**PATIENT:** And I feel, ehm I'm asking too much of the other girls.

**NURSE:** Right.

**PATIENT:** Ehm, if I feel my back's about to go, you know? I can- can't do the moving and handling

**NURSE:** Uh-huh

**PATIENT:** that I should be

**NURSE:** Are you still on the medical ward?

**PATIENT:** doing. Uh-huh

**NURSE:** Gosh, that's heavy.

**PATIENT:** So I've <exhales> I've asked to be moved, in fact, to the clinic.

**NURSE:** Right.

**PATIENT:** Eh, and apparently that's not possible. They want me to stay in the ward. Now, I don't know if there's some kind of sub-text going on there that I'm supposed to stay in the ward because I don't know whether it doesn't suit them to put me in the clinic, or because <exhales> you know I've been there for a long time and I know it all pretty well.

**NURSE:** Uh-huh.

**PATIENT:** Ehm maybe

**NURSE:** Do you think it's because you're a more experienced member of staff, they maybe don't want to lose you?

**PATIENT:** Ah, I think there's,

NURSE: Right.
PATIENT: I think they're a bit reluctant. I mean, having said that, I'm off sick such a lot with this now I'm beginning to wonder why they can't just let me get out of there. But I just, what I want to do is if they won't move me out of there, I'm, I'm going to have to resign.
NURSE: Okay.
PATIENT: I'm going to have to resign. If I have to resign I'm going to, see what really annoys me is, years ago when we were at that nurse training, we were so <exhales> we're so kind of trusting, you know? They showed us this is the way you move and handle patients
NURSE: Mmhmm.
PATIENT: and so I did that, eh and then I hurt myself. And, what I'm, what I'm saying is, I want to, I want to sue
NURSE: Okay.
PATIENT: the health board. Because we weren't taught to move and handle the right way. And I need, I need help with that.
NURSE: Right.
PATIENT: So, what I've come to ask for today is can you help me with this?

The exchange shows the nurse having to deal with a potential conflict: the patient comes to her as both a friend and a colleague, and so the nurse wishes to show both sympathy and professional solidarity. The patient first requests the painkiller, framing the request as a routine response to a recurrent problem, previously sanctioned by her General Practitioner (GP). In her response, the nurse makes her sympathy explicit ('I'm obviously very concerned about your back pain') but points out that she is unable to prescribe the painkiller herself. Instead, she offers a swift consultation with the GP. The patient accepts this alternative, then moves to her second request which she frames at some length: she hurt her back when working on a medical ward; she blames inadequate training; she also blames the administration for not moving her to other duties which would be lighter. She is therefore considering resigning and is requesting the nurse's help in taking legal action against the health board. She presents herself as a victim in this: as a trainee nurse she trusted authority, she cannot understand why she cannot be moved, and her actions are motivated by her concern for her colleagues whom she cannot support as she wishes. The nurse again expresses understanding of the patient's situation ('Gosh that's heavy'), but offers a more positive interpretation of the administration's decision not to move her from the medical ward ('Do you think it's because you're a more experienced member of staff, they maybe don't want to lose you?'). Mostly, however, she listens, back-channelling appropriately ('Right, okay, uh-huh, mmhmmm', etc.) as the patient expresses her problems.

Devising 'critical incidents' such as the above, recording them and analysing the interaction is a typical way of developing strategies for understanding and dealing with a range of difficult or embarrassing situations. The students can role-play the part of patient and nurse or clinician, then reflect on how they dealt with the situation, and analyse in some detail the language they used to cope – here with a difficult request, intensified by the patient's clear appeal to professional solidarity. Simulations are tried and tested means of delivering both medical education and language education though, as we shall see in Chapter 7, they are not beyond criticism.

# Intercultural Interactions in Medical Settings

The present chapter has drawn on only a portion of the extensive research into face-to-face discourse in medical contexts; however, it covers many of the areas that medical students might usefully consider:

- How clinicians communicate with patients from different backgrounds.
- How they communicate with patients in the presence of a care-giver or through an interpreter.
- How junior doctors interact with their senior colleagues.
- How medical professionals might characterise their patients and working conditions informally.
- How non-professionals characterise the medical profession.
- How communication might be made more effective by paying attention to explicit framing of discourse.

In each of these contexts, the intercultural speaker might be expected to develop those *savoirs* that relate to knowing how social interaction occurs, how to interpret and relate information and how to mediate (cf Byram, 1997: 49–54). However, perhaps the most crucial criterion for achieving competence in medical settings is Byram's stipulation that 'the ability to operate knowledge, attitudes and skills' should be demonstrated 'under the constraints of real-time communication and interaction'. Medical interactions are notoriously time-limited and stressful; all the more reason why medical students should have the opportunity for extensive observation and rehearsal in the different settings in which they occur. Through the observation of real-time clinical interactions, or their recordings, role-played interactions in a variety of dyadic and triadic configurations, discussion of drama and literary texts, and mock case studies and examinations, medical students can be encouraged to develop and reflect upon the skills necessary to be an intercultural speaker in a medical setting.

## Notes

(1) A number of transcription conventions are used by different conversation analysts. In this book, we have not attempted to harmonise them; they are retained as they were in the original source documents, with some occasional simplification for reasons of clarity. For a discussion of issues related to transcribing conversation, see Roberts (1997).

(2) See the Connecting Worlds manual and workbook: retrieved from http://www.calendow.org/uploadedFiles/connecting_worlds_manual.pdf and http://www.calendow.org/uploadedFiles/connecting_worlds_workbook.pdf

(3) The authors are grateful for permission granted by KMU to observe and discuss various communicative events in this University and its hospital, including case presentations.

(4) We are grateful to Ms Alna Robb of the School of Medicine, Glasgow University, for allowing us to use this extract from the simulation transcript.

# 6 Critical Cultural Awareness in Medical Education

So far in this volume we have considered the curricular goals of intercultural language teaching in medical education, how intercultural communicative competence might be taught, aspects of the 'languastructure' of medical English, and how face-to-face interaction might be understood in a range of medical settings. The present chapter moves beyond a focused concern for medical language to consider the role of critical cultural awareness in language education for medical students. We cover the following areas:

- How to define critical cultural awareness in intercultural language education for medical students.
- The contribution played by the sociology of medicine and critical medical anthropology in the development of the professional values of 'western' biomedicine.
- Case studies and activities that can be adapted for language classes in medical settings.

## Savoir s'Engager: Critical Cultural Awareness

As we saw in Chapter 2, critical cultural awareness is one of the five *savoirs* discussed by Byram (e.g. 1997, 2008); however, of all the aspects of intercultural communicative competence, it is one of the least defined and most controversial. Byram frames critical cultural awareness in the context of general education at secondary and post-secondary levels, and in doing so suggests that language learners should be invited to reflect on the political nature and implications of their learning. For Guilherme (2002), reflection on the political nature of education leads inevitably to a pedagogy of active citizenship, and the intercultural language classroom then becomes a site for

an open discussion of and intervention in social issues, in the critical pedagogical tradition of educationalists such as Freire (1970) and Giroux (1992,
2001). Risager also links *savoir s'engager* to global citizenship, invoking
Bourdieu's (1979, 1984) notion of 'habitus', that accumulation of 'symbolic
forms of capital that dispose [participants in intercultural encounters] to, or
orientate them towards, particular positions in the cultural encounter'
(Risager, 2007: 234). The intercultural speaker as global citizen will be alert
to the position he or she has been primed to take, and should be able to
'decentre' if conflict arises, and take up the position of mediator.

Byram, Guilherme, Risager and others who write about critical cultural
awareness usually do so from the perspective of general education, often at
secondary school level, and so their guidelines are broadly framed: young
learners should consider the impact their education is having on the formation of their identity, more mature learners should seek to draw on their
education to make a contribution to democratic processes in society and they
should be able to draw on their awareness of different cultural positions as a
resource in situations of conflict. In their introduction to a collection of
papers that aims to link theoretical approaches to intercultural and critical
language education, Phipps and Levine (2010: 6) unpack the concept of 'criti-
cality' in a way that is helpful for language teachers in medical contexts:

> *critical* theory is a means for language program directors, teachers and
> students to unpack, examine and transform assumptions that have
> become so ingrained in curricular, language-program-direction, and
> teaching practices that they are considered second nature.

This call to 'unpack, examine and transform assumptions' resonates with
Barnett's (1994: 108) argument that the critical teacher's role is to act as a
'subversive', lessening the hold that one form of understanding has on the
student, and subjecting his or her assumptions to rational scrutiny (see
Chapters 2 and 3 above). In the context of intercultural language education in
medical contexts, then, the development of critical cultural awareness may
usefully be directed towards means of 'unpacking, examining and transform-
ing assumptions' about the tenets of western biomedical professionalism, the
core set of beliefs that global medical education tends to instil in medical
students. As they go through medical education, students tend to be socialised
into a set of unspoken assumptions about the nature of illness and well-being,
and these very assumptions may hinder effective communication with
patients who do not share their socialisation, or indeed their beliefs. Lay perspectives on medicine may give rise to conflict with the professional view; for
example, a cardiologist may wish to convince a patient to undergo an invasive,

surgical procedure for a deteriorating heart complaint, while the patient may prefer to rely on diet and alternative therapies to manage the illness. The cardiologist may become frustrated with the patient's 'stubbornness' in the face of a worsening condition, and accuse them of being in 'denial.' The break-down in communication can be seen as an intercultural one: the professional values of the cardiologist are in conflict with the lay beliefs of the patient. One may attempt to dominate the other, or they may attempt, through mutual understanding of the perspective of the other, to come to some kind of accommodation – if that is possible. In any negotiation, the values of the professional *and* the lay patient may need to be re-thought and re-aligned for any progress to be made. Neither can afford to be too rigid.

The intercultural language classroom, then, can become a site for subject-ing medical students' professional values to scrutiny, in the hope that some of the more obstructive assumptions might be transformed, or at least that their hold on students might be lessened. The teacher of intercultural com-municative competence in medical settings can draw on several established disciplines to support a challenge to professional biomedical values. Here we consider how insights from the sociology of medicine and critical medical anthropology can stimulate reflection on values in the intercultural language classroom. In Chapters 7 and 8, we extend this discussion further through an engagement with the medical humanities.

# Different Perspectives on Illness and Disease

Since the medical student is learning to become a professional – or to put it another way, is assuming a professional identity – the lay perspective is something that they might readily dismiss as uninformed or even super-stitious. Such an attitude may hinder the construction of a relationship of trust between professional and patient, and cause problems of miscommu-nication. Attitudes about the relationship between professional and patient are often 'unpacked' and the language classroom can be a place for unpack-ing them. For example, medical students can be asked to consider the fol-lowing characterisations of doctors and patients, drawn from different models of medicine and society, namely functionalism, Marxism and social constructivism, in that order (e.g. Lupton, 2003: 5–22). Student can rank the different characterisations of medicine and society in terms of 'truthfulness' and consider how a doctor who adopts one or another perspective might behave in a consultation with a richer or a poorer patient, a man or a woman, a member of the elites or a member of a social minority. The sample activity below can act as an initial step in inviting medical students to reflect on their own 'unpacked assumptions' about their social roles: do they see themselves as benevolent experts, as gatekeepers to scarce medical resources, or as collaborators in the joint production of medical knowledge, a knowledge that is specific to a particular time and place?

## Activity: Examining perspectives on medicine and society

There are different ways of thinking about the relationship of medicine with wider society. Consider the following brief descriptions. Which seems to you to be the 'truest' description of this relationship?

### Perspective 1

Society expects its members to be independent, to work to contribute to the social good, and generally to fulfil their social obligations. If an individual is unable to do that, he or she can be classified as 'sick'. This allows the individual to rely on others, and to avoid work and other responsibilities without feeling guilty. However, the individual is expected to seek help from the medical professions. Healthcare professionals, in turn, have the duty to alleviate the sick person's condition, where possible, so that they can return to 'normality'. The patient is usually the passive recipient of the doctor's expertise and goodwill.

### Perspective 2

Healthcare is a limited and expensive resource. Those who are wealthy or powerful have greater access to healthcare, while poorer or more marginal groups in society have less access, and so their health is poorer. Society, however, needs a healthy workforce. Healthcare professionals are encouraged to focus on the biomedical causes of disease, prescribing drugs and treatment that will sustain the powerful pharmaceutical industry. They are encouraged to neglect the wider social causes of disease, such as poverty, poor diet and a poor living environment.

### Perspective 3

Medicine is a socially situated phenomenon. Many conditions that are diagnosed and treated today would not have been recognised in earlier years; for example, seasonal affective disorder (SAD), or post-viral fatigue syndrome. Other complaints, such as female hysteria, are no longer recognized as medical disorders. When doctors and patients communicate, each draws upon current research, general assumptions, personal prejudices and cultural values to produce a form of knowledge and a joint plan of action that are specific to a particular time and place. No medical knowledge is absolute or universal.

There is some truth in all of the above perspectives, of course, and none alone captures the full complexity of the social role of medicine and medical professionals. Asking students to rank them in their own order of 'truthfulness' will reveal more about their own assumptions than about the actual place of medicine in society, and serve as a first step in critical reflection.

## Power and Authority in Medical Encounters

The first two perspectives outlined in the activity above both assume that the patient has a relatively passive role in the professional–patient relationship. In the first, the doctor is the benevolent expert, guiding the patient back to healthy 'normality'; in the second, the doctor is seen more as an agent of the social elite, administering treatments to alleviate immediate symptoms while neglecting wider social deprivation as a cause of ill health. In each case, the doctor is in the position of authority and power. Students might justifiably feel that, after many years of intensive study and the achievement of a medical degree, they are highly skilled and competent practitioners, whose expertise grants them a legitimate authority in any medical encounter. Indeed, the scepticism that some students report to us about medical communication classes might well have their origins in a challenge to that expertise from outside the medical community. However, it is an established fact from the literature on medicine that patients also have power. Those patients who are in a position to pay for healthcare can, of course, demand a level of service and attention that others may not be in a position to expect. However, even patients from the minorities, also have power of sorts – the power of resistance to hitherto agreed courses of treatment. Lupton (2003: 123) cites a study of Puerto Rican women attending a clinic in the USA (Lazarus, 1988) in which the women commonly resisted medical judgements, procedures or doctors' behaviour they disliked by missing appointments, telling doctors what they wanted to hear and refusing to speak English in subsequent interactions.

As we saw in Chapter 2, much of the motivation for teaching cross-cultural competence in medical education is indeed directed at raising levels of adherence to courses of treatment amongst particular minority groups (e.g. Betancourt et al., 2003). However, a narrow focus on what used to be called 'compliance' may frame the power relationship between doctor and patient in an unhelpful way: patients may be expected to be passively 'compliant' in the face of expertise, authority and institutional power. Those who are not 'compliant' may be seen as socially irresponsible and undeserving of medical treatment, as in the second perspective on medicine and society given above. Stein (1990; cited in Lupton, 2003: 134) unpicks the 'unofficial moral taxonomy of types of patients' shared by medical professionals in one hospital setting: 'good' patients are compliant while uncompliant patients are labelled as 'trolls', 'wimps', 'jerks', 'problem patients,' 'cry-babies' and 'whiners' (Stein, 1990: 71; compare Anspach (1988) and the discussions of doctors' use of derogatory terms in Chapter 7 of the present volume).

An alternative to the notion of the outdated concept of 'compliance' is that of 'trust', a word with a complex history, but whose useful meaning here would be along the lines of 'confidence in and reliance upon the ability, expertise and good intentions of a person.' 'Trust' is built mutually between doctor and patient: the patient must develop trust in the doctor's competence and good intentions; the doctor must develop trust in the patient's responsible response to the treatment they prescribe. Trust is earned over time.

Critical cultural awareness, then, can legitimately raise the issue of what medical students see as a 'good' patient. Again, a ranking activity, such as the one below, can be given as a discussion exercise in the language classroom.

## Activity: Defining the 'good' patient

Rank the following patients in order, from 'good' (1) towards 'bad' (5). Be prepared to justify your opinion.

*Connie* is a quiet Filipino woman, who works as a maid. She attends the clinic and says very little. She does exactly what the doctor advises. She never asks questions and is always grateful for any treatment suggested.

*Jin* is from mainland China. He smokes a lot and refuses to give up. This is not helping his condition. He makes jokes and is very easy to get along with, but sometimes he does what he is told, and sometimes he just doesn't.

*Betty* is a well educated woman from Brazil. She checks out her symptoms on the internet and always has questions when she attends the clinic. If she doesn't understand why the doctor is giving her certain advice, she is not afraid to challenge it. Sometimes she suggests a course of treatment before the doctor does. Once she agrees to an action plan, though, she sticks to it.

*Tony* is from Italy. He is a manual worker and he is not very communicative in the clinic. He says he is following the doctor's advice, but you cannot be sure that he is. He says his English is poor but he seems to understand more than he claims to.

*Theresa* is a wealthy and well educated Turkish woman. She has health insurance and you know that she consults several doctors, including you, about her condition. She seems to listen to several medical opinions and then she chooses the treatment that she prefers.

Different students will no doubt rank the patients differently – an outcome that again should reveal hitherto unpacked assumptions. After ranking the patients as 'good' or 'bad', the students can be asked how they would develop a relationship of trust with each of them. For example, the students might suggest spending a little extra time with 'Connie', asking direct questions about her experience of the treatment she is receiving; time might be taken with 'Betty' to check out how reliable the medical websites she is consulting are; 'Tony' and 'Jin' might be encouraged to reflect explicitly on how their behaviour might be impacting on their health, while 'Theresa' might be asked to reflect on how different suggested courses of action might affect her in different ways. However, trust is not a commodity that can be dispensed like a drug; it is the gradual, earned outcome of a mutual, honest relationship whereby the doctor's expertise guides the patient, and the patient develops a role as a reliable partner in his or her own healthcare. In the development of this role, however, both patient and doctor may have to negotiate their assumptions of what 'healthcare' actually means; the following section explores these assumptions in more detail.

## Curing and Healing, Disease and Illness

In their survey of medical anthropology in a global perspective, Strathern and Stewart (1999) take the title of their volume from a distinction between 'curing' and 'healing', which aligns with a further distinction between 'disease' and 'illness' that some sociologists of medicine also make (cf Kleinman, 1980, 1988; Posner, 1991; Turner, 1996; Lupton, 2003, 93–94). To take the latter dichotomy first, 'disease' refers specifically to the biological complaint, clinically conceived, whilst 'illness' refers to the patient's perception of their impairment in a cultural context. Thus a male teenager's 'disease' might refer to an increase in the production of testosterone following puberty, resulting in the sebaceous glands producing more oily substance, sebum, than is neces-sary to lubricate the skin and hair. The 'illness' would be the teenager's expe-rience of acne, an often an embarrassing and even distressing condition, given the insecurities often attendant on adolescence, the fears of social exclusion, and the strongly positive cultural value given to a 'clear' complex-ion, reinforced by advertising and peer-group pressures.

'Curing', then, relates specifically to the clinical treatment of a disease whilst 'healing' attends to the broader experience of illness as perceived by the patient. As Strathern and Stewart (1999: 7) put it:

> As we, and other medical anthropologists, use the term, curing refers to an act of treating successfully a specific condition, for example a wound or a case of diarrhea or infestation by worms. Healing, by contrast, refers to the whole person or the whole body seen as an integrated system with both physical and spiritual components. Biomedicine, in this view, deals with curing and not healing; alternative medicine and the medical sys-tems of various cultures may depend on a philosophy of healing that either encompasses or stands outside of curing.

As Strathern and Stewart acknowledge, the black-and-white distinction has its limitations: non-Western alternative therapies may also have curing as an aim, while some practitioners of Western biomedicine might also embrace 'alternative' practices such as acupuncture. However, while the distinction between curing and healing may be blurred in practice, it remains a useful interpretive tool for critical cultural awareness in medical education. Essentially, the distinction refers to a narrow focus on the biomedical causes of a condition, which medical training and expertise allow the physician to diagnose, or a wider focus on the patient's experience of a complaint, which the physician then takes into consideration in their treatment. Thus con-ceived, the curing/healing distinction can be used to analyse doctor–patient interactions by considering if and when the physician switches from one mode to the other. For example, once the distinction has been explained to students, they can be asked how the medical student (the resident) and the senior physician (the attending) pay attention to curing and healing in the following scenario (adapted from Strathern & Stewart, 1999: 180–181):

---

## Activity: Healing versus curing

Are 'healing' and 'curing' different processes? Consider the differences between them in the scenario below.

A 54 year-old Native American patient presented at a diabetes clinic for one of her regular check-ups. Her tests at these check-ups consistently showed high blood sugar levels. When questioned about her hyperglycemia, the patient explained that it was caused by anxiety about her 13-year-old daughter's behaviour. She also admitted that she followed her diet plan loosely and ate high sugar food, such as cake, without altering her insulin intake.

The resident recommended increasing the patient's insulin intake in general. When reporting the patient's history to the senior, attending physician afterwards, it became obvious that the resident had based this decision mainly on the patient's chart, and had not paid much attention to the questions and answers. The senior physician suggested discussing with the patient how she might manage her anxiety about her child, whether her 'binges' on high sugar food might be 'comfort eating' as a response to stress, and how she might perhaps regulate her insulin in accordance with her occasionally high sugar intake.

This scenario, like most actual medical situations, is not a problem that has a single or easy solution. The resident in focusing on a 'cure' for the high sugar levels might indeed succeed in treating the patient's hyperglycemia; the senior physician in attempting to attend to the wider social issues affecting the patient would have to depend on the patient's ability to manage her personal relationships and dietary regime more successfully. The patient's expectations would also enter the equation: she may indeed expect the physicians to deal with her problem through medication; she may or may not welcome intervention in her personal affairs, even in the form of supportive advice.

The point of using this scenario, then, is not to arrive at the 'correct' solution to the problem. It is to allow students the space to debate possible ways of approaching the situation; demonstrating the complementary value systems of 'curing' and 'healing' that might inform different ways of treating the patient; and encouraging them to develop a flexible judgement about which set of values to adopt depending on the contexts they find themselves in.

# Medical Pluralism in Japan

The values associated with healing rather than curing may, of course, conflict with the values the professional physician has been trained to accept as part of western biomedical practices. In particular, there is in some quarters a reasoned scepticism about alternative medicines which may be conceived of as superstitious, ill regulated, and even parasitical on the gullibility and fears of uninformed lay people. Such attitudes to alternative medicine are forcefully expressed in Angell and Kassirer's (1998: 841) critique of the use of alternative medicines in self-treatment:

It is time for the scientific community to stop giving alternative medicine a free ride. There cannot be two kinds of medicine – conventional and alternative. There is only medicine that has been adequately tested and medicine that has not, medicine that works and medicine that may or may not work. Once a treatment has been tested rigorously, it no longer matters whether it was considered alternative at the outset. If it is found to be reasonably safe and effective, it will be accepted. But assertions, speculation, and testimonials do not substitute for evidence. Alternative treatments should be subjected to scientific testing no less rigorous than that required for conventional treatments.

An echo of this sentiment can be found in the opening words of an editorial in the *Journal of the American Medical Association* from the same year (Fontanarosa & Lundberg, 1998: 1618)

There is no alternative medicine. There is only scientifically proven, evidence-based medicine supported by solid data or unproven medicine, for which scientific evidence is lacking. Whether a therapeutic practice is "Eastern" or "Western," is unconventional or mainstream, or involves mind-body techniques or molecular genetics is largely irrelevant except for historical purposes and cultural interest.

It is not difficult for the teacher to find similar sentiments expressed in professional medical literature: such views represent a strong ethos in western biomedicine that the focus of treatment should be on curing the disease using scientifically tested and reliable procedures, rather than in healing the illness using methods of dubious value. However, the rational cultural values of the professional physician may come into conflict with the different values and belief systems of patients. While we do not wish at all to diminish the benefits of western biomedicine, we do wish to draw attention to the practical issues that may be raised when the cultural values of professional physicians do not align with those of their patients. Strathern and Stewart (1999: 181–182) go so far as to suggest that medical professionals should have a veritable constellation of resources to draw upon if they wish to communicate effectively, and heal as well as cure:

> Attempting to understand the whole patient and treat the whole person who exists within a complex social nexus is one of the more insightful ways of lessening communication problems. Biomedicine needs to draw upon cosmology, ontology, epistemology, understandings of personhood, society, morality and religion for its most effective expression.

Medical anthropologists have suggested that, in many cultures, pluralist or syncretist approaches to healing are the norm rather than the exception (Stoner, 1986). Stoner and Strathern and Stewart cite Lock's (1980) study of *kanpo* clinics in urban Japan, where biomedically-trained physicians, sometimes wearing white coat and stethoscope, practise alternative medical approaches, based on an understanding of well-being as a balance and harmony. As Strathern and Stewart (1999: 24) observe, drawing again on Lock (1980):

> Several factors are involved: *Kanpo* has come to stand for "Japanese culture"; it is recognized for insurance purposes; and it is an agreeable therapy for older patients with long-term chronic conditions who can make frequent, almost social visits to herbal clinics; and above all the herbal regimen suits Japanese ideas of the body and its needs. Biomedical treatment is seen as invasive and aggressive, especially in the form of surgery, whereas herbal medicines are seen more as foods, nourishing the body and helping to restore the balance of substances within it.

The notion of 'balance' is clearly central to alternative medical systems like *kanpo*. Worsley (1982) cautions against 'over-systematising' folk medical beliefs; however, he acknowledges that many are based on humoral oppositions (hot versus cold, wet versus dry, bitter versus sweet etc. Reflecting on these oppositions, in the medical culture of the Nahua, an indigenous Central American people, Worsely (1982: 318) further comments that:

> Structuralist anthropology would simply observe that hot/cold is a primordial, available opposition, like masculine/feminine, likely to be seized upon as something good to think with; ready-made, universal and archetypal elements of human existence with potential as categories for ordering the world, whether for dividing it into the feminine tables and masculine blackboards of the French, or the hot ice-creams or conceptually "hot" meat of the Nahua (even when it is physically cold).

Long-established humoral categories permeate lay discourse about health, then, even when those who use the terms are unaware of the 'system' that lies, or once lay, behind them. For example, a Brazilian patient may avoid chocolate as a 'hot' food when they have a fever; a physician may consider this an uninformed opinion, or alternatively as something to take into consideration and work with constructively when advising the patient more generally on dietary options to manage or relieve the condition.

In an intercultural language course for medical students, the issue of medical pluralism can be raised, again, to challenge the set of values associated with so-called 'western' or 'professional' biomedicine. The purpose of raising this issue would not be to set alternative medicine against more or less superior 'scientific' practices, but to explore how best to communicate with patients whose view of medical treatment is at least partially informed by traditional beliefs about health, which may indeed extend into areas of morality and religion. The following activity may be used to initiate classroom discussion.

---

## Activity: Exploring beliefs about health

Are you familiar with any of the following popular sayings or beliefs about health? Do you know any others? Are any popular with your family members?

*An apple a day keeps the doctor away.*

*To cure warts, rub them with a potato and then bury the potato. Say a prayer.*

*Feed a cold, starve a fever.*

*Hypertension is caused by 'thick blood'; eat bananas or drink passion-flower tea to cool the blood.*

*Taking ginseng is good for the memory.*

*Apple cider vinegar helps cure arthritis.*

As a physician, (a) how would you find out whether your patient was using any of these or other 'folk remedies', and (b) how would you react if you discovered that the patient *was* using the remedy?

As people who are becoming professional physicians, medical students may adopt the attitude expressed by Angell and Kassirer (1998) or Fontanarosa and Lundberg (1998), quoted above, that alternative, humoral or 'folk' remedies are useless, untrustworthy and possibly even dangerous, unless subjected to rigorous scientific scrutiny. However, when negotiating an action plan with a patient, the physician may have to set aside this attitude and investigate the patient's belief system in order to arrive at a mutual agreement about the treatment. In many situations around the world, healing, as opposed to curing, involves a pluralistic view of medicine in which both western biomedicine and alternative perspectives play complementary roles – the most remarkable example probably being *kanpo*.

# The Healthcare Professional as Ethnographer

Strathern and Stewart's stricture, quoted above, that the effective physician needs to draw upon resources not only from biomedicine but from disciplines stretching from cosmology to religion may be over-ambitious, or at least daunting for the medical student who is already struggling with the wealth of information to be absorbed from biomedical training. One possible way of addressing this problem is not for the medical student to know about all these disciplines, but for him or her to be prepared to learn about them, through observation and questioning. Effectively, the medical student, like the intercultural language student, can be encouraged to become a practical ethnographer (cf Damen, 1987; Roberts *et al.*, 2001; Corbett, 2003: 94–117). Ethnographers develop systematic means of observation and interview in order to be able to describe and interpret the cultural codes and rules underlying individuals' behaviour in communities. Damen's (1987: 63, 64–69) advice on doing 'pragmatic ethnography' – that is, ethnography directed towards 'personal and practical purposes and not to provide scientific data and theory' – can be adapted for use by medical students who wish to supplement their clinical case histories with a broader instrument for exploring patients' cultural beliefs:[1]

(1)  Describe your patient: age, gender, ethnicity, social class, and so on.
(2)  If your patient is part of a particular social group (e.g. Asian, Hispanic, etc.), do some library research to investigate whether she is likely to be familiar with an 'alternative' medical system. However, do not make assumptions that she practises or believes in such a system.
(3)  In your case interview, elicit from the patient how she understands her complaint and how she might be self-treating by asking questions such

as: 'What do you think might have caused your condition?', 'Most of us have favourite remedies for treating different illnesses. Are you doing anything to treat this condition?' and 'Are members of your family giving you support, or advice about how to deal with your illness?'
(4) Be careful not to make evaluative comments in response to the patient's replies. If the patient indicates use of folk remedies in the management of her illness, you might suggest other such remedies, so long as they are not incompatible with the recommended treatment. For example, a Hispanic patient who is taking fluids to treat a virus might be advised to drink camomile tea (a common folk remedy for anxiety and nausea). The integration of biomedical advice and folk remedies can in certain circumstances build up a relationship of trust between the professional physician and the patient.

Over time, and with the experience of treating different patients from different cultural backgrounds, the ethnographer-physician should build up a working knowledge of different kinds of lay medical belief system. Of course, the medical student who has yet to accumulate these layers of lived knowledge should not fall into the trap of stereotyping, for example, all Hispanic or Japanese patients as believers in folk remedies or alternative medical systems like *kanpo*. Writing of the cultural complexity of the USA, Betancourt (2003: 562) cautions:

Traditionally, cross-cultural education has focused on a "multicultural," or "categorical," approach, providing knowledge about the attitudes, values, beliefs, and behaviors of certain cultural groups. For example, methods to care for the "Asian" patient, or the "Hispanic" patient, would present a list of such patients' common health beliefs, behaviors, and key practice "do's and don'ts." With the huge array of cultural, ethnic, national, and religious groups in the United States, and the multiple influences, such as acculturation and socioeconomic status, that lead to intragroup variability, it is difficult to teach a set of unifying facts or cultural norms (such as "fatalism" among Hispanics or "passivity" among Asians) about any particular group. These efforts can lead to stereotyping, and oversimplification of culture, without a respect for its fluidity. Research has shown that teaching "cultural knowledge," when not done carefully, can be more detrimental than helpful.

As noted above, some knowledge of an individual's *possible* culturally-influenced attitudes, values, beliefs and behaviour in relation to lay medical practices can be useful to the physician in eliciting information about the patient's *actual* attitudes, values, beliefs and behaviour. But the intercultural medical student needs to use observation and the opportunity for cultural exploration afforded by the case history interview to explore how the individual patient positions herself with respect to the complex 'fluidity' of cultural influences in a globalised and multicultural world.

## Illness and Metaphor

We conclude this chapter with two brief case studies that extend the discussion of critical cultural awareness beyond 'alternative medical systems,' as such, and towards more general cultural conceptions of illness, gender and medical professionalism. The foregoing sections counterbalanced the biomedical value system that physicians are normally socialised into with lay, folk or alternative medical belief systems that patients draw upon. Our argument is that rather than dismissing alternative perspectives as irrational and unscientific, as intercultural speakers and listeners, physicians might take the opportunity to explore them with their patients, coming to a 'third place' (cf Kramsch, 1993) where the biomedical and lay perspectives on medicine might positively complement each other. This process of attaining a 'third place' involves students in subjecting their own value system, and those of others, to critical scrutiny, to the point at which a transcendent perspective is possible. Critical cultural awareness, however, can extend beyond medical systems to a consideration of how society at large expresses concepts relevant to medicine and to those who are receiving medical support.

In an influential polemic, Susan Sontag (1978) drew on her own experience as a patient with breast cancer to explore the impact that stereotypical depictions of 'master illnesses' like tuberculosis and cancer had on those suffering from them. Revisiting the topic in a later volume (1989), she extends her argument to the then recent AIDS epidemic, and recalls the motivation for writing the earlier book. Her thesis is that certain diseases are invested with social meanings, through art, literature, advertising, and other public discourses, that often terrify or stigmatise their sufferers, preventing some from seeking support from the medical profession, and demoralising others to an extent that may inhibit recovery. Sontag (2002: 98) writes:

> As tuberculosis had been often regarded sentimentally, as an enhancement of identity, cancer was regarded with irrational revulsion, as a diminution of the self. There were also similar fictions of responsibility

and of a characterological predisposition to the illness: cancer is regarded as a disease to which the psychically defeated, the inexpressive, the repressed – especially those who have repressed anger or sexual feelings – are particularly prone, as tuberculosis was regarded throughout the nineteenth and early twentieth centuries (until, indeed, it was discovered how to cure it) as a disease apt to strike the hypersensitive, the talented, the passionate.

Sontag's two volumes remain influential and compelling although some of the attitudes she expresses might now appear dated, and, indeed, in the second volume she acknowledges that metaphorical thinking is a crucial means by which we understand our world. Seen as personal documents from the 'front line' of suffering, they can be read as attempts to counter the myths and metaphors attracting to stigmatised diseases, spotlighting, for example, the military metaphors that are used in the 'battle' or 'fight' to 'kill' an 'aggressive' disease; and the ways in which cancer is generally used as a metaphor for 'an event and situation that is unqualifiedly and unredeemably wicked' (Sontag, 2002: 83), and usually incurable except through invasive surgery that cuts the tumour out. Examples taken from a search for *cancer* in the *Time* magazine corpus over the course of the 20th century include the following (http://corpus.byu.edu/time; see Chapter 4 for further information about corpus searches):

> In the April number of Columbia, the Knights of Columbus magazine, Mr. Justice Joseph Morschauser (also of the New York State Supreme Court – who presided at the Stillman case and other divorce suits) advocated the abolition of divorce in the United States. "Divorce," said he, "is a **cancer** in the vitals of American life .... From my experience on the bench I know that halfway reforms are ineffective. The only way to cure the evils of divorce is to completely abolish divorce." (*Time*, 31 March 1923)

> Fuchs is a type of traitor which the U.S. has recently and reluctantly come to recognize. It is the type of the intelligent, talented, apparently sincere man who suffers from Communism's moral **cancer**, the man who can calmly do wrong and pretend to himself that he is doing right-because in his mind he has obliterated right and wrong. (*Time*, 20 February 1950)

> he rebuilt his frame into something sleeker and better suited to pedaling up mountains. He came back to the Tour last year looking as skeletal as **cancer** itself but then dominated both the mountains and the individual time trials. "I lost all the muscle I ever built up, and when I recovered, it

didn't come back in the same way," he wrote in his book *It's Not About the Bike*, published last month (Putnam; $24.95). (*Time*, 24 April, 2000)

While we can see in the first two examples in particular the kind of metaphorical use of 'cancer' against which Sontag argues, it is clear from the searches of the *Time* corpus that literal uses of the word are far more frequent than metaphorical ones in the magazine. Indeed, in the 2000s, it becomes more difficult to find metaphorical uses of that characterise something morally evil as a 'cancer', the final example being the non-literal personification of cancer as death, in an article about a cancer sufferer who went on to recover and regain his status as a competitive cyclist.

In the intercultural language classroom with medical students, reading passages from literature, advertising and political and news broadcasts can alert learners to the ways in which certain diseases have been and continue to be characterised in popular culture (for background, see Priscilla Wald's (2008) study *Contagious*, which makes a fascinating counterpart to Steven Soderbergh's later film, *Contagion*, 2011). Literature, art and other forms of the media, too, can be used to sensitise students to popular representations of disease in society, and their possible impact (see further, Chapters 7 and 8). Martin (1991) and Lupton (2003: 74–75), for example, draw attention to metaphors for reproduction in popular science genres such as television programmes and educational explanations. Despite biomedicine's descriptions of an active ovum, popular representations of medicine often personify the 'masculine' sperm as the active agent, undertaking an arduous journey through the vagina and up the fallopian tubes, to where a passive, 'feminine' ovum is awaiting union, coyly and patiently. Martin (1991: 498) suggests that the stereotypical masculine/feminine metaphors that popular science draws upon in its descriptions of reproduction and fertility have consequences in debates about the role of medicine in regulating reproduction, through abortion, contraception, artificial insemination and genetic screening. Similarly, Wald warns of the power of popular 'outbreak narratives' to frame the ways that non-professionals, medical scientists and healthcare policy-makers think about disease and disease control: she argues that by personalising diseases with human characteristics, by focusing on a few affected individuals and by diverting resources to investigate possible mechanisms by which contagions such as typhoid and AIDS were carried by those individuals, other means of disease control, which focus on systemic causes and issues of social justice, might be neglected (Wald, 2008: 270; see further, Chapter 7).

The motivation to explore the metaphoric portrayals of illness and disease is similar to the motivation to address alternative medical systems. By considering other ways of thinking about familiar issues, medical students are encouraged to subject their own attitudes and values to rational scrutiny. They may emerge from this process with their beliefs confirmed and strengthened, or they find their core values qualified. Either way they will have become reflective thinkers, and so demonstrated aspects of their intercultural communicative competence.

## Birth in Different Cultures

As we have seen so far in this chapter, intercultural language education encourages learners to learn about the behaviour, attitudes, beliefs and values of people in different communities, whether these communities are defined in terms of professional versus lay groups, or in national or ethnic terms. In medical education, developing the *savoir* of critical cultural awareness might include comparing learners' attitudes to general medical topics, such as birth, across different countries. The management of pregnancy and childbirth has varied considerably over time as well as geographically, as Lupton (2003: 159) observes in some detail:

> Since the late nineteenth century, pregnancy and childbirth have become progressively medicalized and the pregnant woman cast as a patient. While hardly any women received prenatal medical care in the United States in 1900, by the end of the century almost all received such care regularly. Over that time in the medical literature, pregnancy became portrayed as more pathological and pregnant women as therefore requiring close medical surveillance (Barker 1998). There is currently a lively debate about the necessity for having all births attended in hospital, and the safety of home births.

The sociology of medicine thus portrays childbirth as a site of struggle and control: who is the prime agent with responsibility for delivering the child – the mother, the midwife or the physician? How is power and authority distributed amongst the participants involved? What, if any, is the role of the father, or other family and friends, at the moment of birth? These issues are indeed lively, and so useful for stimulating debate in intercultural language classes for medical students, where attitudes across cultures, genders and the lay/professional divide can be explored.

Current institutional attitudes to birth in Britain are expressed, for example, in the UK National Health Service's advice to pregnant women, given on the NHS Direct website (see Figure 6.1). Various assumptions and points for negotiation are evident in this advice.

---

**What is a birth plan?**

It's a written record of what you would like to happen during your labour and after your baby's born.
If you think beforehand about the options you might face, you can decide what you would prefer
before you go into labour.
Around week 34 of your pregnancy, your midwife or GP will give you information about preparing
for labour and birth, including developing your birth plan.

**What should I include?**

Your birth plan is personal to you. It will depend on:

- what you want,
- your medical history, and
- what's available at your maternity service.

Your birth plan can include information such as:

- where you'd like to give birth (at home, in a midwife unit or hospital),
- who you'd like to be with you,
- what position you'd like to be in during labour,
- whether you want pain relief and, if so, your preferred choice (such as pethidine, epidural, or gas and air),
- if you want an injection to speed up delivery of the placenta, or if you want it to be natural,
- how you feel about an assisted birth or caesarean section if things don't go to plan,
- where you would like your birth partner to stand, for example, at your head,
- if you want your baby placed straight on your stomach before they are cleaned,
- how you plan to feed your baby (breastfeed or bottle feed), and
- whether you agree to having student nurses, midwives or doctors present.

You should also include any special requirements, for example:

- you or your partner have special needs, such as wheelchair access,
- you need someone present who speaks your first language,
- you need a special diet while you're in hospital, or
- you wish special religious customs to be observed.

You'll probably want to think about or discuss some things more fully with the baby's father and
friends and relatives.

---

**Figure 6.1** Writing a birth plan (NHS Direct)[2]

The NHS birth plan might be used to raise the following points in the
language class:

- In other countries, is there an equivalent of the 'birth plan' recommended
  for pregnant women in the UK?
- What degree of control should patients themselves have in the 'manage-
  ment of [their] childbirth experience'? In particular,
  - Who should be present at the birth?
  - Who should decide delivery position?

- ○ What music – if any – should be played?
- ○ Who should make decisions about methods of pain relief?
- ○ Who should cut the umbilical cord?
- ○ Where should the baby be placed after birth?

The NHS advice is culturally interesting from several perspectives. First, it acknowledges that the delivery of the child is not the only aspect of the service that the NHS should provide. Rather, giving birth is part of a complex experience that may be shared by a 'birth partner', and may be marked by religious rituals. The negotiation and distribution of responsibility for decision-making, between mother, birth partner and professionals, is a key feature of advice given to birth partners on other websites, such as Babycentre UK's '10 tips for labour partners', which includes the advice given in Figure 6.2.

Note that the NHS advice and the Babycentre UK's advice do *not* provide factual information about how women actually give birth in the UK. They do, however, reveal some of the issues about the values and beliefs that inform behaviour in the birth room. Namely, in the UK it is accepted that generally birth partners – who may not always be the husband – have a role to play that might be both practical and symbolic. It is also accepted that mothers have a considerable degree of responsibility for aspects of their healthcare during labour; and sometimes the birth partner acts as the mother's advocate and guarantor of her wishes during the period of labour.

The services and procedures offered to women and their partners during childbirth in different countries may or may not be similar to those currently offered in the UK, but clearly practices do vary from place to place and from time to time. In Russia in the 1980s, fathers were discouraged from visiting hospitals during labour and for 10 days thereafter, for reasons of 'sanitation'. A Russian novel by Julia Vosnesenskaya, *The Women's Decameron* (1987) is a series of stories told by women who are confined in a maternity home for the 10 days of their 'quarantine'. Other cultures illustrate other customs and

---

*Know your limits*

There's a lot going on in the birth room. Be aware of what you are willing to do during the process, and what you want to leave to the professionals.

Mathew remembers the midwife asking if he wanted to catch his son when he came out. "I decided not to as I was worried about doing it," he says. "But I did cut the umbilical cord. That was easy."

---

**Figure 6.2** From 'Dads: 10 ways to be the perfect birth partner' (Babycentre UK)[3]

beliefs: in Chinese communities, for example, there are various constraints on the mother's diet and behaviour in the first month after childbirth. They should refrain from washing their hair; they are expected to avoid cool air and cold foods; recommended food includes chicken soup with some Chinese herbal medicine added. Texts from different countries can therefore be used to display different attitudes, values, beliefs and behaviours. In terms of the *savoirs* that guide intercultural language education, the NHS and Babycentre UK advice websites can be used to explore:

- The relationship of the individual to society (here, the relationship of the pregnant mother and her partner to state institutions such as the National Health Service).
- How interaction occurs (via a written 'birth plan' and the spoken advocacy of the mother and her birthing partner).
- Critical cultural awareness (considering who has responsibility for healthcare decisions and when).
- Knowledge of how to discover cultural information (healthcare consultations, websites and leaflets, but also television and film dramas, novels, etc.).
- Empathy – why is it important for childbirth to be a whole 'experience' for all involved, from mother to doctor, midwife and birthing partner?

From this example, it is evident that an intercultural language curriculum for students of medicine could include topics and texts that address aspects of healthcare practice such as birth, the care of terminally ill patients, or the stereotypical image of 'the doctor' or 'the nurse' across cultures, and consider critically how the texts articulate social values, attitudes and beliefs, and how these, in turn, inform behaviour.

The present chapter has moved from a discussion of critical cultural awareness in the intercultural language classroom, to illustrations of how comparisons between 'biomedical' and 'alternative' medical systems might challenge students' implicit or explicit socialisation into the 'professional' medical values espoused by scientific medicine. We have suggested that the distinction made by medical anthropologists between 'curing' and 'healing' might inform approaches that accept medical pluralism in an attempt to negotiate a 'third place' between professional and lay perspectives of medicine. To find this 'third place', medical students might usefully add the tools of practical ethnography to those of taking a clinical case history. We have looked briefly at how popular representations of high-profile illnesses in society might adversely affect patients suffering from those diseases, and suggested ways in which medical educators might follow Sontag (2002) in 'demystifying' these culturally-loaded images by drawing critical attention to them. And, finally, the case of childbirth in different cultures and times was offered as an example of how longstanding debates in medical practices can cast light on issues of gender, authority and agency.

This chapter, then, has moved us from a focus on competences and teaching practices (Chapters 2 and 3) and the nature of medical language and discourse (Chapters 4 and 5) towards a critical exploration of values in language and medical education. The following chapters, 7 and 8, continue this exploration by discussing what the medical humanities might offer to intercultural language learning for medical students.

## Notes

(1)  This section also draws on Nancy Neff, M.D.'s module on folk medicine in the Hispanic American community, available online at http://www.rice.edu/projects/HispanicHealth/Courses/mod7/mod7.html [Accessed June 2011].

(2)  Source: http://www.nhs.uk/chq/Pages/2296.aspx?CategoryID = 54&SubCategory ID = 135 [Accessed 24 September 2011].

(3)  From http://www.babycentre.co.uk/pregnancy/labourandbirth/planningyourbabys birth/labourpartnerstips [Accessed 24th September 2011].

# 7 Literature and Language in Medical Education

Chapters 7 and 8 explore the roles that the medical humanities, in particular literature and the visual arts, can play in raising issues to be addressed by English language teachers working in medical contexts. The humanities – which now generally include subjects such as literature, media studies, philosophy, history and art – have long played a central role in general education, and increasingly the medical humanities have become a fixture in the training of healthcare professionals (e.g. Evans & Finlay, 2001; Skelton 2000a, 2000b). Much of the focus of the medical humanities in the UK has been on history, with scholars such as MacNeill (1979), Porter (1999, 2005) and Cohn (2010) discussing the interaction between disease, medical thinking and society in general. Increasingly, the topic of medicine has become of interest to literary and media scholars and students (e.g. Hawkins & McEntyre, 2000; Harper & Moor, 2005). Literature, in turn, has always had a lively if volatile place in the English language classroom (e.g. Carter & Long, 1990; Lazar, 1993; MacRae, 1991; Hall, 2005) and its use in intercultural language education, alongside media and cultural studies, is briefly discussed in Corbett (2003: 166–190).

The present chapter focuses first on some of the reasons for including the medical humanities in intercultural language education for medical students. We then turn to resources and the design of suitable tasks for literary analysis, discussion and reflection. In the following chapter, we extend the discussion to include the visual arts, including film and television. In many respects the division between the two chapters is arbitrary, and it is of course fruitful in many educational contexts to integrate the study of literature and the visual arts – indeed, film and television are obviously hybrid art forms, combining dramatic scripts with dynamic visual compositions. However, we devote separate chapters to the two domains since language teachers often have more experience of literary education, and the techniques of analysing and discussing the visual arts are often less familiar.

## Why the Medical Humanities?

The claims made for the value of integrating the humanities in medical curricula are diverse in nature and are subject to debate (e.g. Evans & Finlay, 2001; Shapiro *et al.*, 2009). The humanities are generally held to encourage the following attributes and activities:

* the development of the 'whole person';
* the development of ethical standards;
* the empathic identification with people of different social and cultural backgrounds;
* practical skills of observation, analysis, reflection and critical thinking.

It is worth spending some time considering these claims. The study of the medical humanities is often credited with supporting the development of the 'rounded human being' or 'whole person', indicating an anxiety that purely instrumental medical education fails to inculcate desirable values in trainee healthcare professionals. Shapiro (2006) notes that courses in the medical humanities and arts have been offered in medical education in 50–75% of all North American medical schools. The goals of such curricular are various, as noted above, but generally speaking, include:

> a desire to educate medical students and residents more broadly about the human condition; help them to understand different points of view and thus to develop clinical empathy; stimulate reflection and critical thinking; better tolerate ambiguity and uncertainty; and reconnect them with aspects of awe and mystery in the practice of medicine. (Shapiro, 2006: 3–4)

The fact that there is a perceived need for courses to 'reconnect' medical students with the 'awe and mystery' of their profession speaks to a general social anxiety about the 'dehumanised' nature of healthcare. Goulston (2001: 123) gives voice to this anxiety, suggesting that doctors are perceived as 'over-materialistic, lacking the qualities of caring and compassion, and unable or unwilling to communicate adequately with patients'. The 2003 edition of *Tomorrow's Doctors* (General Medical Council, 1993, 2003, 2009), a set of guidelines designed to shape the curricula offered in UK medical schools, explicitly differentiates 'education' from simple 'training'. The document argues that 'education' provides a more holistic cultivation of tomorrow's doctors and makes explicit the fact that clinicians will frequently experience intercultural encounters, not only with patients from different countries (GMC, 2003: 17):

A medical student is supposed to know the social and cultural environment in which medicine is practiced. They are expected to understand a range of social and cultural values, and differing views about healthcare and illness [...] They must recognize the need to make sure that they are not prejudiced by patients' lifestyle, culture, beliefs, race, colour, gender, sexuality, age, mental or physical disability and social or economic status.

The most recent edition of the same document (GMC, 2009: 21) is more succinct in its recommendation that tomorrow's doctors should be able to:

Communicate clearly, sensitively and effectively with individuals and groups regardless of their age, social, cultural or ethnic backgrounds or their disabilities, including when English is not the patient's first language.

The growth of medical humanities across the globe may be seen as a response to the perceived need to educate clinicians to be 'sensitive' and thus 'effective'; the integration of the humanities into medical education is intended to 'enrich a narrow curriculum that was focused, almost exclusively, on the value-neutral transfer of scientific fact' (Hunter et al., 1995, cited in Goulston, 2001: 125).

Incorporating the medical humanities into medical education also draws on the long history of the humanities in addressing values; the subjects that make up the humanities all provide a discursive space in which students can discuss issues of belief, values, ethical awareness and ethical standards. In Taiwan, for example, the humanities are taught in the initial part of a 7-year medical degree to encourage medical students to 'learn to be human before learning to be a doctor' (Huang, 2002:134). However, Friedman (2002: 321) provides a useful corrective to any tendency for the humanities to claim a monopoly – or even a special place – in the teaching of ethics and values in medical education:

As now conceived and taught in most medical schools across the country, bioethics should not be considered to be part of the medical humanities, and certainly should not be sanctioned as such within the curriculum. To do so represents a significant mistake, because bioethics and the medical humanities, as widely taught within the same academic health care programs, represent distinctly different ways of analyzing information, viewing the world, confronting dilemmas, and teaching students.

Friedman argues cogently that there is room for both bioethics and the medical humanities as distinct parts of an admittedly crowded medical education curriculum. The former discipline has evolved into a means of enabling clinicians to adhere to ethical standards and deal with moral dilemmas in their professional lives; the latter has a broader function: to allow clinicians space for reflection on their emotional and affective responses to their medical experiences, and on the place of their profession in wider culture. Literature, in this scheme, has its place in part because it allows clinicians to confront emotional issues and debates relating to their personal and professional identity at a 'safe' remove. Charon (2000: 29) makes the case for literature more strongly:

> Teaching literature to doctors and medical students fulfils embarrassingly instrumental goals at the same time that it allows wild conceptual play. Instrumentally, training in such literary concepts as genre, narrative stance, reader response, subtext, metatext, and imagery can provide medical students and doctors with skills that their elders did not have, never got and did without. Patients have suffered long enough the consequences of a medicine practiced by doctors without these skills – doctors who cannot follow a narrative thread; who cannot adopt an alien perspective; who become unreliable narrators of other people's stories; who are deaf to voice and image; and who do not always include in their regard human motives, yearnings, symbols, and the fellowship born of common language.

In language education in medical contexts, of course, the 'fellowship born of common language' is less of a given. Literature, however, has long enjoyed a place in language education, even if, relative to the claims sometimes made for the value of the humanities in medical education, those made for the particular utility of literature in the language classroom are modest. Hall (2005: 48) summarises them as:

- motivating learners, giving pleasure;
- giving access to cultural and intercultural knowledge;
- practice in discourse skills such as inferencing, dealing with ambiguity, and so on;
- vocabulary enhancement;
- developing reading fluency;
- developing interpretative skills;
- promoting the use of memory.

Hall (2005: 48) further notes that while many of these claims are well grounded, they are too often 'taken on trust', and the same might be argued for the more general claims made for the role of the humanities in medical education. It is true that the processes by which clinicians become 'well rounded,' 'whole' or 'empathic' people are still under-researched. Even so, we can argue that the humanities offer curricular space in which educators and students can raise issues of value, emotion, and cultural difference, and explore aspects of interculturality. They may also practise observational skills, analysis, reflection and critical thinking. As noted above, one major virtue of literature is that 'it provides a means of attending to voices other than those presented in habitual social and professional situations' (Collett & McLachlan, 2006: 59). The value of literature in medical education, for both older and younger readers, then, is in part that it extends their world experience beyond the familiar, that it provides access to different cultural communities – whether defined by class, generation, ethnicity, race or national belonging.

The arguments in favour of literature teaching in medical and language education resonate strongly with intercultural language education. Reading and studying literature encourage a 'decentring' from one's own perspective, confront readers with alternative value systems, and invite both an emotional response and a reflection on that emotional response. Literature speaks to most of Byram's *savoirs* (see Chapter 2); for example, it invites openness about other belief systems, which may be dramatised in the literary text; reading literature demands different interpretative strategies; the content of literary texts might broaden the readers' knowledge of different social groups; and, again, literature may invite critical reflection on different cultural practices.

## Resources for Teaching the Medical Humanities

There are many printed anthologies that focus on medicine and literature (e.g. Bamforth, 2003) and a number of recommendations of literary texts that deal explicitly with medical issues (e.g. Ho, 2003; McEntyre, 2000; Salinsky, 2002). McEntyre includes in her list of 'medical standards' the short stories 'The Use of Force' by William Carlos Williams (Coles, 1993: 56–60) and 'Indian Camp' by Ernest Hemingway (Hemingway, 1966: 89–95), as well as the novels *Cancer Ward* (Solzhenitsyn, 1968) and *The Citadel* (Cronin, 1937), the plays *Angels in America* (Kushner, 1992, 1993) and *The Elephant Man* (Pomerance, 1979) and some non-fiction. Writing in a non-Anglophone context, Ho (2003) recommends that Taiwanese doctors read *The House of God* (Shem, 1979), *A Fortunate Man: The Story of a Country Doctor* (Berger &

Mohr, 1967) and *The Diving Bell and The Butterfly* (Bauby, 1997) alongside
local Taiwanese literature. The textbook, *Doctors in Fiction: Lessons from
Literature* (Surawicz & Jacobson, 2009) presents and discusses the fictional
representations of more than 30 physicians, while the compilation *On
Doctoring* (Reynolds and Stone, 2001) collects a wide selection of fiction,
poetry, and even a complete play, all with a medical theme. A glance at these
various volumes shows a possibly disturbing recurrent theme: as Salinsky
(2002: 4) observes, doctors in fiction frequently show 'a dismaying lack of
moral fibre, decency, or even professional competence'. As Skelton (2000a:
1921) also observes, doctors in literature, like their counterparts in film and
television, tend to be poor role models for medical students (compare the
discussion of *Grey's Anatomy* in Chapter 8); however, for this very reason,
fictional texts make for good classroom discussion.

Relevant texts may be selected from such anthologies and recommendations because they deal directly with the experiences of health professionals or patients, but this need not be the main criterion. It is true that
the literary 'touchstones' recommended by McEntyre (2000) might provide
medical practitioners with professional insights or topics for discussion.
Medical memoirs such as Gabriel Weston's *Direct Red* (2009) can 'prompt
reflection on aspects of professional life, such as what to do in moments of
panic, how to deal with conflict, how to cope with an error of judgement,
and so on' (Lu & Corbett, 2010: 84–85). Short stories such Hemingway's
'Indian Camp' (Hemingway, 1966), in which a young boy accompanies his
physician father to a Native American reservation, where the father will
assist in a difficult birth, raises issues pertinent to medical practitioners,
such as the dangers attending middle-class professionalism and the objec-
tification of the patient in situations of physical and mental suffering on
the part of both patients and their families. However, texts that are not
primarily concerned with medicine can be usefully exploited; for example,
Marshall and Bleakley (2009) use a famous scene in Homer's *Illiad* in which
Andromache, the wife of Hector, pleads with him to stay within the city
walls of Troy and not to go to the fight with Achilles, to initiate a discussion of how pity in Homer can be transformed into empathy in medical
education.

A major online resource for teaching the medical humanities is the New
York University website (http://medhum.med.nyu.edu/) which includes a
database of a wide selection of literature and the visual and performing arts
that can be used to stimulate discussion in medical education. The items in
the database are annotated with summaries and commentaries that indicate
their potential interest to medical educators. For example, the database annotation for Ernest Hemingway's 'Indian Camp' is given in the box below; the

summary and commentary may themselves form a starting-point for class-room discussion of the story.

---

**Summary**: From a fishing trip the local doctor is summoned to an Indian village to assist a woman in labor. With him are his young son and an older male relative. The physician assesses the situation in the closed, pungent hut and determines that his only option is section— with a pen knife and fishing leader as his instruments, and no anesthesia for the Indian woman. The doctor arrogantly, but only briefly, celebrates his success as a surgeon only to discover that the woman's husband, apparently unable to tolerate his wife's pain and the racism of the white visitors, has silently slit his own throat. The child, who has observed the entire proceedings asks, "Is dying hard, Daddy?"

**Commentary**: This very short, terse piece from Hemingway's Nick Adams stories is laden with ethical problems. What justification is there for forcing a child to become part of a brutal sequence of medical events? When, if ever, is it morally acceptable to treat patients as though they were animals? The medical treatment of the laboring woman is unquestionably life-saving, but the cruel insensitivity of the two white men contributes to the unnecessary death of the infant's father. Duties to children and to patients, as well as simple inhuman-ity, racism, and sexism in the professional relationship are all aired in these five pages.

---

Source: http://litmed.med.nyu.edu/Annotation?action=view&annid=795

Anthologies, annotated databases and even scholarly essays, however, may not be sufficient guidance for the teacher wishing to use literature or the visual or performing arts for intercultural language education in the medical curriculum. The following section of this chapter illustrates princi-ples of text selection and task design for the use of medical humanities mate-rials in the intercultural language classroom.

## Selecting Appropriate Texts

The selection of appropriate resources for medical education will depend on the goals of particular curricula and classes. Some texts might indeed be chosen because of their direct relevance, because they offer a dramatised instance of typical real-life situations. For example, the dialogue between the character Ray Cohn and his physician in Tony Kushner's *Angels in America* can be used to discuss the issues raised by hostile patients who resist a stigmatising diagnosis (see the brief discussion in Chapter 5). The activity below picks up on another theme noted in Chapter 5, namely some physicians' habit of referring to patients using derogatory terms, and uses a fictional illustration to open discussion on the implications of naming practices.

## Activity: Medical slang

Samuel Shem's comic novel, *The House of God* (1978) follows a fictional intern through a traumatic first year, in which he is introduced to a range of technical and slang terms, many of which are listed in a glossary at the end of the novel. His most reliable guide to the subculture of the hospital is another character, the Fat Man, who introduces the narrator and his junior colleagues to the language of the discipline, including the term *gomer*, which describes elderly patients suffering from dementia (Shem, 1978: 37; adapted).

Read the passage and consider the following questions:

(1) Have you ever heard medical staff use slang like this?
(2) Have you used this kind of slang yourself? If so, in what kind of contexts?
(3) In the following passage, whose point of view is closest to your own, that of Potts or The Fat Man ('Fats')?
(4) How important is it to pay attention to the kind of language that is used to describe patients, both in professional and informal settings?

'Gomer is an acronym: Get Out of My Emergency Room – it's what you want to say when one's sent in from the nursing home at three A.M.'

'I think that's kind of crass,' said Potts. 'Some of us don't feel that way about old people.'

'You think I don't have a grandmother?' asked Fats indignantly. 'I do, and she's the cutest, dearest, most wonderful old lady. [...]'

I thought of my grandfather. I loved him too.

'But gomers are not just dear old people,' said Fats. 'Gomers are human beings who have lost what goes into being human beings. They want to die and we will not let them. We're cruel to the gomers, by saving them, and they're cruel to us, by fighting tooth and nail against our trying to save them. They hurt us, we hurt them.'

This extract from *The House of God* can prompt a classroom discussion that might also be informed by sociologists' analysis of non-fictional doctors' use of derogatory slang – and other, less obviously dehumanising naming practices. Anspach (1988) acknowledges that sociologists studying this phenomenon in the latter part of the 20th century found it difficult to understand trainee physicians' use of a slang terms that so obviously demean the very people they are trying to care for. Shem's novel problematises the issue by showing that the verbal denigration of elderly patients is not necessarily incompatible with care; indeed, some sociologists have argued that it is a necessary 'safety valve' for trainees who are developing a necessary emotional distance from the everyday traumas they have to deal with. However, Shem's novel also acknowledges the dehumanising aspects of the socialisation of young clinicians into the medical professional community. Anspach (1988) picks up on this theme, and broadens it out to a wider range of contexts, showing, for example, how medical students use a set of linguistic strategies in case presentations to distance and depersonalise the human encounter between physician and patient. In particular, she focuses on the following features of professional discourse, written and spoken, in case presentations:

- the separation of biological processes from the person (de-personalization);
- omission of the agent (e.g. use of the passive voice);
- treating medical technology as the agent;
- account markers, such as 'states,' 'reports,' and 'denies,' which emphasize the subjectivity of the patient's accounts.

Using a fictional example of 'doctor talk' can be a relatively non-threatening means of initiating discussion of the ways language creates, sustains and reinforces a set of attitudes towards patients.

The example from *The House of God* focuses on a specific aspect of medical life and discourse. Other literary materials may be selected to encourage more general transferable skills, such as observation and deduction. Listening to patients, taking case histories and doing presentations and seminars are how doctors 'tell stories' (Calman, 1997; Salinsky, 2002). Charon (2005, 2006, 2007) uses narrative fiction and poetry to develop medical students' expertise in reading, attentive listening, reflective writing and bearing witness to suffering.

Overall, then, the selection of literary materials in the medical humanities will be determined by their value in:

- giving insight into professional practice and ethical dilemmas;
- extending practitioners' experience of different communities and cultures;

- offering case studies for observation, discussion and diagnosis;
- reflecting on and enhancing general skills such as empathy and critical thinking.

# Task Design: Medicine, Literature and Intercultural Language Education

In Chapter 3 we argued that task design for the intercultural language classroom in medical contexts differs little in principle from that devised for the general language classroom as described, for example, by Nunan (1989, 2004), and that it bears many resemblances to problem-based learning in medical education. Applications of task design to literature in the language classroom are discussed in detail by Lazar (1993). The teacher who wishes to use medical humanities learning materials should, at minimum, consider the following issues, again based on the task format discussed in Chapter 3.

## The goals of the task

- Is the task designed to encourage, say, observation of a medical condition, or to initiate class discussion of a problematical situation or difficult ethical dilemma?
- Is the task designed to address an aspect of intercultural or cross-cultural communication; for example, to encourage re-evaluation of a stigmatised community; to probe stereotypes; to stimulate critical thinking; or to heighten awareness of a particularly difficult communicative situation, such as the delivery of bad news to a hostile patient from an unfamiliar community?
- Is the task designed to enhance a particular set of language skills, such as knowledge of vocabulary, fluency in reading or speaking, formal presentation of information etc?

## The input

- What is the nature of the input, for example, poem, short story, novella, script, painting, sculpture, installation, television programme, film, theatrical production?
- What kind of linguistic demands does the input make on the learner? How might these be lessened, for example, by preparation or contextualisation, pre-teaching of key vocabulary, and so on?

## Activities

- What kind of response might the input normally evoke, for example, retelling, paraphrase, completion, speculation, description, comparison, explanation, evaluation?
- Can the classroom activities draw upon these 'normal responses'? To what extent are these 'real world tasks' (e.g. a 'diagnosis' based on a literary text might mirror a 'real world' diagnosis; the discussion of ethical procedures in a novel might take the form of dinner-table discussion between professional colleagues).
- To what extent can the activities be broken down into 'subskills' of language use? For example, Nunan (2004: 62–63) draws on Lai's (1997) inventory of reading skills, the most salient being:
  - ○ having a clear purpose for reading;
  - ○ previewing the text;
  - ○ skimming and scanning;
  - ○ predicting the outcome;
  - ○ inferring ideas and meanings;
  - ○ identifying figurative expressions;
  - ○ using background knowledge;
  - ○ identifying style and its purpose;
  - ○ reading critically;
  - ○ integrating information;
  - ○ reviewing the text.

Does the classroom activity target these reading skills and does the teacher support them?

Lazar (1993: 127) suggests a three-stage approach to designing activities for reading literature: (i) pre-reading activities to familiarise students with context; (ii) while-reading activities to deal with issues of language; (iii) post-reading activities to explore responses, debate themes, etc. What kind of activities would you select for each stage of the literature task?

## Settings

As we saw in Chapter 2, learning activities may be accomplished in different settings. Increasingly, language learning tasks may occur outside the conventional environments, spilling over from the classroom to the workplace, the home, or – increasingly, with online intercultural exchanges – to the virtual environment, via electronic communications (e.g. Warschauer & Kern, 2000; O'Dowd, 2007; see further, below). Project work might take learners to reading groups or literary events. Each space again has its advantages and disadvantages: the conventional classroom has the advantage of the teacher as immediate support and facilitator; the workplace has direct relevance to the learners' professional lives; virtual environments (such as on-line reading groups) add the spice of 'real communication' but without, perhaps, the immediately available guidance of a teacher or the richness of face-to-face interaction.

## Teacher's and learners' roles

The 'role' is the set of responsibilities and contributions teacher and learners are expected to make in the design and achievement of the task. Conventionally, teachers may choose goals, select inputs and devise procedures for the learners to carry out individually or in pairs or groups; however, if there is sufficient space in the curriculum, the learners may gradually take more responsibility for choosing the texts and issues that they wish to share and discuss.

## A sample task: 'His son's big doll' by Chun-Ming Huang

This sample activity illustrates how a piece of short fiction may be used with a group of medical students, in this case pre-clinical students at Kaohsiung Medical University in Taiwan. The students tend to be fairly young, and from relatively affluent, urban backgrounds (Fan *et al.*, 2007). The narrow social strata from which medical students are drawn may be perceived as potentially limiting their experience of 'otherness'; literature can therefore function as one way of broadening that experience. In the early part of their seven-year medical curriculum, the literature classes are based on broad themes such as 'the individual and society'. Specific readings are selected for their potential in evoking empathy, pity and compassion, and the opportunity they provide for observation, analysis, comparison, reflection and critical thinking. The texts chosen included William Faulkner's 'A Rose for Emily', Chun-ming Huang's 'His Son's Big Doll' and Edwin Arlington Robinson's 'Richard Cory'. Here, we illustrate the issues raised by tasks relating to Chun-ming Huang's 'His Son's Big Doll'.

The goals of the reading task were to:

- raise awareness of disadvantaged social groups within the community, particularly the rural community;
- defamiliarise local culture by reading a Taiwanese story in English translation;
- compare interpretations by local students with readings by non-Taiwanese students, via an online reading group;
- reflect on the kinds of domestic pressures that might be faced by socially disadvantaged people who present as patients.

According to commentators such as Thiong'o (1986) and Ho (2003), the use of local literature in English can increase students' engagement with texts and their content, and so one text chosen as input was by Chun-ming Huang, a Taiwanese representative of *hsiang-t'u wen-hsueh*, or 'nativist literature,' a movement that focuses on the lives of rural people, and others who live on the periphery of modern Taiwanese society. In the story, 'His Son's Big Doll', translated and published in the anthology *The Drowning of an Old Cat, and Other Stories* (Huang, 1980), an uneducated man, Kun-shu, living in a Taiwanese suburb in the 1960s, struggles to maintain both his family and his self-esteem. However, employed by a local cinema to advertise movies, dressed as a clown and using a sandwich-board, he loses his sense of self-esteem and, ultimately, his identity, both in his community and at home. The story poignantly dramatises the battle between dignity and survival.

The teachers' and learners' roles in this task were relatively conventional: the teacher set up the reading activities (pre-, while- and post-reading, as outlined below) and the learners accomplished them, drawing on the teacher for support where necessary. In 2010, however, the activity was enhanced by the presence of the author, Chun-ming Huang, at Kaohsiung Medical University, to take students' questions about his work.

The settings for the reading activity blended conventional and online environments (cf O'Dowd, 2007). The medical students generally have better receptive than productive skills, and lack confidence, fluency and accuracy when speaking and writing. The engagement with international co-participants in a reading group, therefore, had the additional goal of prompting the Taiwanese students to extend their writing skills through asynchronous discussion with their online partners. The initial activities were rehearsed by the pre-medical students in the classroom; then the learners' contributions were posted online, prompting responses and further questions from students taking non-medical classes in other countries, in this case the UK and Argentina.[1] As a pre-reading activity, the Taiwanese learners were asked to post a brief outline of Taiwanese history, to contextualise the story for the international participants. The medical students were then asked to read the short story, focusing on the following questions:

- What do you know about the period and the location of the story?
- Does the story give an accurate picture of Taiwanese society: family relationships, work, living conditions?

They then posted their answers to these questions, and the post-reading activity was to discuss the story with their online partners. For their part, the international students were asked to discuss the story in small face-to-face groups, and then post questions to the Taiwanese medical students. An example of a medical student's post in response to the while-reading activity is given below (Figure 7.1).

Here we see one student drawing on family memories as an empathic resource to understand the difficulties faced by rural workers in 1960s Taiwan. Although the students themselves generally form part of an 'elite' in contemporary Taiwanese society, their family and friends may share knowledge of more difficult times and harsher social circumstances; literature can evoke this shared knowledge. When the international students began posting questions, the Taiwanese students were put in the position of acting as cultural informants, explaining aspects of their own society and culture that seemed 'other' to the western participants in the exchange (Figures 7.2 and 7.3). In one case, the question targeted aspects of non-western medicine.

The online reading group incidentally, then, stimulated a discussion about non-Western medicines that displayed a range of attitudes amongst the

> The story is based on the Taiwan society in 1960s. And it was the time that economy just began to grow up. Because there were so many people uneducated, like Kunshu, it is pity that they had to work in the labor level without other ways.
>
> ※ Does the story give an accurate picture of Taiwanese society: family relationships, work, living conditions?
>
> Yes, it did. My father was born in 1940s, and he always says that it was a really hard time for most Taiwan people. The social conception is quite conservative in family, relationships, and work also. So people might not accept fresh things at that time. Thus the "sandwich man" even couldn't be a "job". Family, also, was "traditional", means that men had to work outside, and women did the whole housework. Therefore men felt more pressure while working and the only women could do was to support her men.

**Figure 7.1** Example Taiwanese medical student's post

> [...] the story describes two adverts on his board: "the one in front proclaimed the virtues of Hundred-Herb Tea; the one behind plugged a tapeworm medicine." Is this an indication of the use of herbal remedies in Taiwan? If there is a tradition of this, is it supported in hospitals or is it seperate from the Taiwanese healthcare system? In the UK, herbal remedies are fairly popular however not offered by the NHS, a patient must purchase them privately and a doctor won't recommend them officially.

**Figure 7.2** UK student's question about 'His Son's Big Doll'

> People in Taiwan usually uses herbal remedy to cure the patient, but it is not common in hospitals. It is trational [*sic: traditional*] remedy, so it is common in country.
>
> ***
>
> Actually, Chinese gives priority to traditional Chinese herbal medicine originally. After Western medicine was introduced, however, Chinese began to overthrow the traditional Chinese herbal medicine and even thought it was ridiculous and lack of scientific knowledge. Recently, we found that many diseases (especially chronic disease) are incurable in Western medicine but curable in traditional Chinese medicine, so now people start to examine traditional Chinese medicine which was made by scientific methods.
>
> ***
>
> Herbal remedies play an important role in treating sickness, especially to the elderly. They believed that herbal remedies are the most temperate therapy and would do fewer side effects to human body than medicine. As a result, the healthcare system is surely to support it.

**Figure 7.3** Sample medical students' responses

Taiwanese medical students, including the awareness of a conflict between western biomedical values ('even thought it ridiculous') and a broad sympathy for alternative practices, especially amongst 'the elderly'. The literary text can therefore initiate a broader discussion of professional and non-professional values (cf Chapter 6).

The use of an online reading group, which encourages learners from different backgrounds to explore each other's cultures and preconceptions, gives learners an additional reason for reading literature, particularly local literatures. The Taiwanese medical students were exploring social 'otherness' in their own culture, by reading an English translation of a story that addresses human problems in a period and social class of which they had no direct experience. But, for the international participants in the group, the Taiwanese medical students were privileged cultural informants; and so the medical students were put in the position of explaining details of the story from the perspective of an 'insider'.

# Monitoring Student Responses and Developing Literary Skills

Boyle (1986: 200) suggests that literature is a major resource for language learning because it is 'human nature in action'. Asking learners to keep diaries

Although at the beginning of my reading, I felt a little bit difficult and the ending of the story made me surprised and frightened. However, a while later, I can feel great sorrow flowing in my heart. ... In brief, I really learn a lot from this article.

\*\*\*

William's dad crying in the night is the most touching part (that day William's parents had a fight because of the poor living condition) ... Being poor may not be an experience for most of us, and reading others' experiences is a good way to remind us to cherish what we have and sympathize the poor.

**Figure 7.4** Extracts from learner diaries by Taiwanese medical students

about their responses to the literature they read, or interviewing them individually at certain points during the course, gives the teacher some insight into their developing reflections on human experience as constructed by the texts they are reading. Figure 7.4 gives sample responses by the Taiwanese medical students to other literary texts they were asked to read during their General Education language course.

The sophistication of the responses is, of course, limited by the students' proficiency in English; nevertheless, they still manage to exhibit awareness of the purpose of using literature in medical education. A similar capacity for self-reflection is evident in more proficient student responses to a short story by Thomas Mann, 'The Black Swan' (Lahtinnen & Torppa, 2007). Here, one student reader considers how his or her understanding of a character in the story has been shaped by his or her professional development (Lahtinnen & Torppa, 2007):

I wonder how I would have seen the story if I had read it before my medical studies, or if I had studied psychology instead. Perhaps I wouldn't have been so inclined to link Rosalie's behaviour with her increased hormonal production, but have thought that it was her desire for youth that made her fall in love. That she fell ill with cancer was just an unhappy event, as sudden deaths usually are. The author doesn't give us the answer. For me it is important to think of this question and not to forget its human and non-medical aspects. In medicine we have a tendency to think very logically and to seek causal explanations.

Even in this brief response, we can see some hints of the four key elements that Charon (2000, 2006) suggests that literature can contribute to an understanding of medicine: frame, time, plot and desire. Narratives are *framed* both by the narrator (who might indeed offer a story as a narrative of love) and the reader (who here 'medicalises' the story as a narrative of 'increased hormonal production'). For Charon (2000: 34), readers should be trained, too, to pay attention to *time*, 'the temporal flow of the narrative – structured as it may be in flashbacks, premonitions, backward tellings, and the like – and to discriminate between how the events occurred and how one learns about them in the text.' In a narrative apparently composed of a non-chronological jumble of happenings, it is often the clinician's responsibility to identify the *plot*, that is, a meaningful, ordered sequence of related events, by, as the student puts it in the quotation above, thinking 'very logically' and seeking 'causal explanations.' And finally, as Charon reminds us, and the student clearly understands, patients' stories are about *desire*: what for the student is a clinical problem is, for the character in the story, a consequence of her 'desire for youth'. Paying attention to these aspects of any literary text, and comparing them to non-literary texts such as medical case histories and hospital death summaries, can aid a programmatic approach to the study of literary language in medical settings. For advanced second-language learners, a broader set of systematic strategies for reading literary texts can be developed with reference to the topics covered in a number of good textbooks on the subject (e.g. Montgomery *et al.*, 2007; Thornborrow & Wareing, 1998), for example, narrative point of view, realism, irony, parallelism and the representation of speech and thought.

As we noted above, Charon (2000: 39) makes considerable claims for medical students who acquire proficient literary skills. She concludes:

> When our students learn to approach the clinical stories that they write and read and hear with responsible literary practices, their knowledge of patients and of disease grows in accuracy and depth. As a dividend to themselves that is also a bonus to their patients, they grow in self-knowledge. Because they become good readers, they become good doctors.

Even if the case for a direct relationship between literary and medical skills is made rather forcefully here, we can nevertheless grant a valid place for literature in a language curriculum aimed at medical students. Crucial to both literature and medical practice are sensitive interpretive skills and an attention to the emotional impulse driving patients' narratives. Literary texts are not, however, the only means of developing interpretive skills; neither are they the only arena for discussing ethical issues, values and emotion. In the following chapter, we therefore turn to other and related art-forms that can be of use in language education for medical students: the visual arts, film and television drama.

## Note

(1)  The authors are grateful to the participants in the 'Intercultural Connections' project for granting permission to quote their postings anonymously.

# 8 The Visual Arts in Medical Education

This chapter extends the discussion in Chapter 7 to explore the uses of the visual arts – from painting and conceptual art to medically-themed films and television series – in language classes for medical students. Here, we cover the following issues:

• The uses of visual images in language and medical education.
• Approaches to the teaching and learning of 'visual literacy' with medical students who are undertaking English language courses.
• Some case studies of painting, conceptual art and filmed or televised drama that may be used in the classroom.
• Resources for using the visual arts in language courses for medical students.

In general, the use of the visual arts, film and television in medical education falls, like literature, history and other arts-based disciplines, into the domain of the medical humanities. Therefore there is a considerable overlap between the concerns of the current chapter and that of the foregoing one, which focuses on literature. Many programmes in medical education combine literary, historical and visual materials, to provide a rich stimulus for medical students to raise broader issues about medical issues than are generally addressed by clinical courses. For example, Prewitt (2000) describes a course on 'teaching the body' that includes anatomical illustrations, short fiction, excerpted long fiction, cultural theory and poetry. A beautifully illustrated book on the history of medicine worldwide (Anderson *et al.*, 2011) draws on the resources of the Wellcome Collection to show how artists and scientists from different cultures have mapped the body, understood illness and developed cures, conceptualised the mind and mental illness, and sought to stay well. The volume juxtaposes microscopic images of DNA, drugs, cancer cells, syphilis and the HIV virus with paintings and sketches of medical procedures and conditions, advertisements for health products, and photographs of protective amulets, anatomical sculptures and ritual masks. Similarly, the New York University Medical Humanities Database mentioned in Chapter 7 (http://medhum.med.nyu.edu/) is a rich source of visual materials that can be used in language courses for medical students. While those who use literary and visual materials with students might share common goals, the skills used in the description and interpretation of visual artefacts are in some respects different from those used in literary analysis – although other aspects are analogous and various concerns (e.g. with narrative) may be shared. The present chapter, then, can be read as a complementary continuation of the foregoing one.

## Images in Language and Medical Education

As language teaching handbooks such as Wright (1990) and Goldstein (2009) demonstrate, there is a long and durable tradition of using visual images in language education. Images can provide a focus and context for many students, and teachers are adept at using them to practise targeted language, from descriptive statements to more speculative discussions about past and future (e.g. 'What can you see in the foreground/background?' 'What has just happened?' 'What do you think will happen next?'). Corbett (2003: 139–165) extends such uses of images in the language classroom by incorporating elements of the developing discipline of 'visual literacy' (e.g. Kress & van Leeuwen, 1996). Visually literate readers treat images as culturally constructed messages which represent particular points of view. By paying attention to the cultural construction of images, learners address one key *savoir*, namely 'knowing how to interpret and relate information'. Strategies for developing this aspect of students' visual literacy are summarised below, drawing largely from Corbett (2003), but applying the techniques particularly to images with medical themes. If, as we suggest, visual images can be read as 'messages', then these messages also exist in complex cultural and cross-cultural relations to their producers and consumers, as we demonstrate below with reference to a painting that portrays an iconic – and contested – episode in the encounter between Asian and Western medical practices and religious beliefs.

Medical educators, like their language teaching colleagues, have also recognised the power of visual images to encourage their students to develop observational skills that may include but normally go beyond diagnostic training. Kubetin (2002) reports on a study by Dr Irwin M. Braverman, a professor of dermatology at Yale University, whereby students visited the Center for British Art, and there studied fine art portraiture in some detail in order to develop their observational skills. In tests, they later outperformed a control group of students who either learned more generally about the works of art in the museum, or took a course in taking medical histories (Dolev *et al.*, 2001). In an interview (Kubetin, 2002), Braverman makes the following argument:

"It's easy for us to tell medical students to 'look for the details,' but we have not taught them how to do it until now," he said. The time spent closely observing paintings helps medical students overcome their tendency to ignore the details of familiar things, such as human faces. The human brain censors the details of familiar objects and notices only the most grossly abnormal changes, he said.

In contrast, when someone looks at an unfamiliar painting, all of its details have equal priority. "Censoring by the brain does not automatically occur. This low threshold [for observing detail] is transferable to the physical examination," Dr. Braverman said.

This small-scale experiment suggests that close, systematic attention to painting can accelerate students' development of clinical observation skills. However, most medical programmes that incorporate visual art into their programmes do so for broader reasons, and with a wider range of media than portraiture. Boisaubin and Winkler (2000), for example, argue that engagement with classic and contemporary paintings and advertisements, as well as film and television series, can increase medical students' awareness of the complexity of their patients' 'life contexts'. They describe the development of a two-year component in visual arts at the University of Texas Medical Branch in Galveston, which includes an element on 'life cycles', part of which engages the students in images of pregnancy and motherhood. They advocate using images from different times and places to interrogate the ways that the 'ideal' mother has been culturally constructed, from early paintings of the Madonna, through photographs, to contemporary advertisements (Boisaubin & Winkler, 2000).

Artists may also work directly with medical students. Lu (2010) interviews a conceptual artist, Christine Borland, much of whose work explores medical themes; for example, 'Simulated Patient' is a video installation that directly confronts the difficulties of preparing medical students to break bad news. Borland spent time teaching in Glasgow University's Faculty of Medicine, discussing her work with students and challenging their values and preconceptions – and those of their educators. Some of Borland's work is discussed further below. While many teachers have a background in literature, fewer have enjoyed the benefit of similar training in the visual arts. The following section, then, is devoted to giving some basic guidance in acquiring the 'tools' of visual literacy, through some case studies of how visual materials can be used in language education in medical contexts.

# Developing Visual Literacy

The content of an image has been likened to its vocabulary, while its composition has been likened to its grammar (e.g. Kress & van Leeuwen, 1996). In other words, the composition of an image is an analysis and description of the *arrangement* of the content. An understanding of the visual message takes into consideration the content, the arrangement of the content, and the relation of the image to the viewer. Following Kress and van Leeuwen, Corbett (2003: 160–164) provides a checklist of questions that can be used to 'interrogate' visual images. Not all are applicable to every image, but they represent a place to start when analysing images. The list is adapted below; where they are not reproduced in the text, many of the images referred to are available and annotated in the New York University Medical Humanities Database, or they are accessible via other internet browsers.

(1) *Images of people*
    What kinds of people are shown in the image? Do the characters portrayed conventionally represent any particular values (e.g. the doctors who appear in the American artist Norman Rockwell's early 20th century magazine illustrations tend to be white, male, middle-aged and kind).[1]
(2) *Who or what are the characters looking at?*
    The direction of the characters' gaze and the expressions on their faces indicate their feelings. The observers in Rembrandt's celebrated *The Anatomy Lesson of Dr Nicolaes Tulp* (1632; Figure 8.1), are all male, bourgeois citizens and medical students of the time. They have gathered to watch the public dissection of an executed criminal. Their gazes are directed in different directions: the anatomist's gaze, like many a lecturer's, seems to go over the heads of his audience. Several observers crane their neck to peer closely at the dissected arm. One looks away, towards the textbook on the lower right. Others gaze raptly at the anatomist, apparently intent on his words, and yet another oversees the scene as a whole. In medical education, this painting can be used in different

ways, for example it can prompt reflection on medical students' early experiences of human dissection (Chan & Shum, 2011). An article in the *Journal of Hand Surgery* (Ijpma *et al.*, 2006), discusses the contemporary restaging of the dissection, an event that showed the limits of Rembrandt's nonetheless considerable anatomical understanding. The use of this image is discussed at greater length below.

(3)  *How close are the characters to you?*
Are the characters represented in close-up, medium-shot or long-shot? Are you, as a viewer, intimately involved in the action or are you a distant observer? Are the characters facing you, or angled away from you? Are they addressing you directly, in a friendly, inviting or threatening manner? Are you looking up at the characters or down at them, or are you at eye-level with them? How does your position make you feel about the characters – superior, respectful or equal?

Using the Rembrandt painting (Figure 8.1) again as an example, the viewer is able to look at the anatomist and cadaver, and at his audience. Tulp's own medical textbook is close at hand, to the viewer's right. The scene is viewed from a slight distance, and the viewer looks dispassionately down at the assembly, rather like the audience member in the background. This is an event that has been composed for our benefit: we are privileged observers.

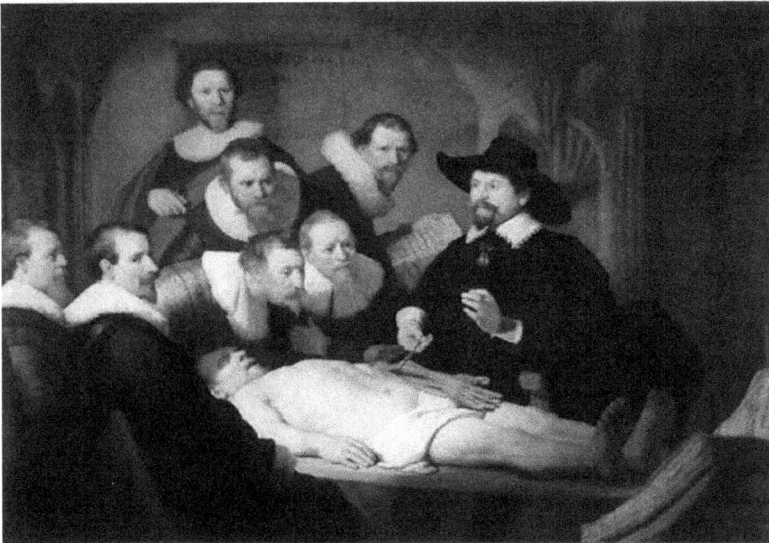

**Figure 8.1** *The Anatomy Lesson of Dr Nicolaes Tulp* by Rembrandt

(4) *Fashion and style*

How are the people in the image dressed, and what does their style of clothing suggest about them? Contemporary paintings of doctors and healthcare workers will often represent them in uniform – doctor's white coat or nurses' uniform. As noted, Norman Rockwell's doctors, when not white-coated, are usually well groomed, be-suited middle-aged males who are often in the company of children (see, e.g. 'Doctor and Doll,' 'The Family Doctor' and 'Doctor and Boy Looking at a Thermometer'). In each case the doctor's clothes show him as a respectable, paternal, presumably trustworthy, middle-class professional, whose concern is to make his young patients feel at ease. The anatomist and observers in Rembrandt's painting are also male and bourgeois, but dressed in dark finery to acknowledge the social importance and solemnity of the occasion of the public dissection.

In fine art, women are more evident as patients than as doctors. In a famous painting *Un Leçon Clinique à la Saltpêtrière* (1887) by André Brouillet (Figure 8.2), the French clinician, Jean-Martin Charcot, stands, like Nicholaes Tulp, lecturing to a large group of black-suited male colleagues and students. But instead of a male cadaver, the object of study is a hypnotised, female 'hysteric', known as 'Blanche', who is portrayed in partial undress, her lace corset revealed and her shoulders bare. She

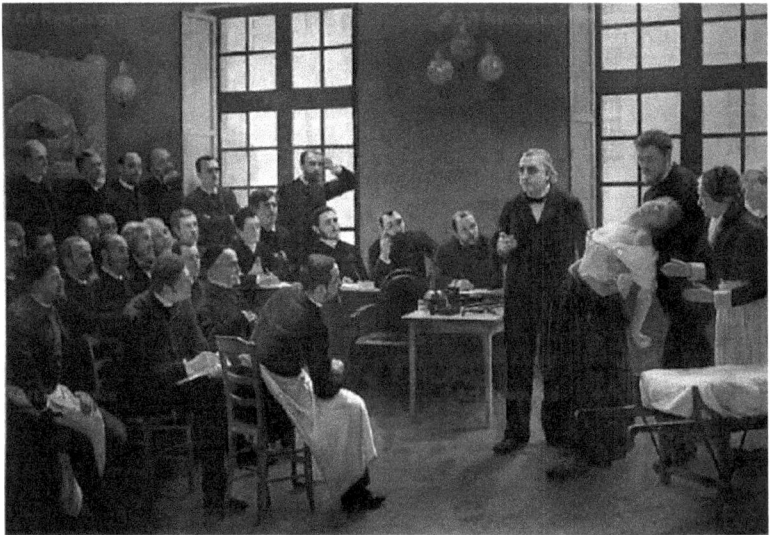

**Figure 8.2** *Un Leçon Clinique à la Saltpêtrière* by André Brouillet

seems unconscious, and is supported by another male – the only other females in the painting are uniformed, older women who stand behind Blanche, ready to catch her if she falls. Here the medical gaze becomes problematic: the young woman, whose white corset contrasts sharply with the sober black suits of the observers, appears to be an object of erotic contemplation for the audience and, by extension, the viewer. In this image, the inevitable voyeurism of the medical demonstration is made explicit and gendered.

(5) *Objects*

Are any objects shown in the image? If so, what are their functions? Can you see all of any object or just part of it? Are you looking from above, below, or head-on? What feelings are the objects intended to evoke; what associations do they have for you? Are you supposed to want or desire the object? Is it associated with any of the characters shown? Does the object have symbolic value? If so, how did it come to have that value? Is that value universal or localised in a particular culture or set of cultures?

In medical images, medical instruments and accessories are clearly associated with the profession. Norman Rockwell's doctors have stethoscopes and thermometers, and they carry voluminous leather bags; in Rembrandt's painting the textbook on display on the lower right-hand side of the painting is a frequent fixture in early anatomical illustrations. In Brouillet's painting (Figure 8.2), on a table behind Charcot, there are various scientific instruments. All the objects depicted, from Rockwell's stethoscope and the big doctor's bags to the glass bottles on the table in Brouillet's painting, suggest scientific knowledge, and thus the authority and power of the medical profession. Without that authority, the actions of anatomists and psychiatrists would be deeply disturbing, even criminal. As the Brouillet painting suggests, even *with* that authority, the actions of clinicians are open to critical appraisal.

---

## Activity: Beginning a visual analysis

Find one or two images of a medical procedure (e.g. by browsing the New York University Database at http://medhum.med.nyu.edu/)

(a)  Describe the kind of people shown in the images.
(b)  Describe who or what they are looking at.
(c)  Consider how the viewer is positioned in relation to the characters portrayed.

(d) Describe the clothing worn by the characters: what does it suggest about them?
(e) Describe any objects shown in the image: suggest their significance.

(6) *Settings*
The characters and objects portrayed in many images are located in a setting. Is the setting identifiable? If so, what is it: urban or rural, public or domestic, familiar or strange, an ocean or a desert? Would you like to be there?

Is there no apparent setting (are the characters or objects shown against a dark or indistinct background)? If there is no identifiable setting, are you therefore being asked to focus on the characters and objects – and if so, why?

Does the setting have any particular associations; for example, the clinical setting of a hospital; the academic setting of a lecture theatre; the spiritual setting of a church or temple?

Is the setting an accurate representation of the place it portrays, or is it romanticised or caricatured? If the setting is a partial representation of a particular place, why do you think *this* setting has been chosen?

The paintings discussed thus far (Figures 8.1 and 8.2) again serve as examples of different artistic choices. Rembrandt's painting of Tulp and his audience has a dark, relatively indistinct setting; the lecture hall is dimly lit with crypt-like arches and a poster is sketched in the background. The lighting draws the viewer's gaze to the central cadaver, the artist and the circle of observers. By contrast, Brouillet's painting is set in the brightly-lit, identifiable location of a lecture theatre in the Saltpêtrière hospital, a site whose dry, academic respectability is at odds with the eroticised subject of the doctor's lesson. Norman Rockwell's doctors are typically depicted in rural clinics or idealised family homes in small-town America; they represent paternalistic care in communities that exist on a human scale.

(7) *Composition*
Kress and van Leeuwen (1996: 208ff) suggest that there are conventional meanings to the arrangement of elements in any visual image. These conventions are culturally shaped, but in images that are influenced by western traditions, the placing of elements in the image is influenced by diverse factors, such as the direction in which we read and the long history of religious art. In centre-dominated images, important content is placed at the centre while less important content is placed at

the margins. Idealised content may be placed in the upper part of the image (the conventional site of heaven in western religious art), while realistic content is placed in the lower part. In left-to-right-dominated images, the content on the right tends to be new or salient, and should be interpreted in relation to the content on the left, which contextualises it.

If we return to the painting of Nicolaes Tulp's anatomy lecture, the central image is that of the cadaver, with the focal point being Tulp's hand, using scissors to raise the body's exposed left arm to public view. The arrangement of cadaver, clinician and audience draws the viewer in as a participant in the public dissection: the viewer is positioned as a fellow member of the audience. In Brouillet's painting, however, the clinician and his female patient are situated on the right-hand side of the frame, contextualised by the lecture audience on the left. The viewer is not part of this audience, but looks on the scene from a detached and critical perspective. In Kress and van Leeuwen's terms, since they are situated to the right in the field of view, the doctor and patient in Brouillet's image constitute the salient or new content, to be interpreted here as objects of the audience's curious and voyeuristic gaze. The female patient is situated farther to the right than the doctor, and so, the visual grammar suggests, her role may be understood in the context of the clinician's lecture.

(8)  *Framing*

When looking at the contents of an image, we can ask whether the elements are shown as a whole, or whether they are separated by some kind of 'frame'. The frame can be a line, formed by part of the setting (e.g. a window or doorway), by something someone is holding, or by changes in lighting or shadow, or colour. In Rembrandt's painting of Tulp's anatomy lecture, the members of the audience are shown as a homogenous group, arranged in a circle under one of the arches of the lecture hall. As we noted above, they are also dressed similarly, with sober suits and wide, starched, ruff collars. Tulp himself is separated by being under a different, smaller arch; his clothes are darker, his lace collar is more modest and he is wearing a large wide-brimmed hat. The cadaver lies brightly-lit on the table; however, the upper part of the face of the executed criminal is shaded by the body of one of the observers: the dead man's face is the only one in the painting that is partly shadowed. In this image, while the observers, anatomist and cadaver are all distinguished in some way (by shadows, by clothing and by position with respect to the arches of the lecture hall), the overall framing suggests one composed scene. The brim of Tulp's hat and the grouping of the observers parallel the arches of the lecture hall, and the viewer's eye is swept around the scene as a single whole.

By contrast, in Brouillet's painting of Charcot's lecture, the tall windows divide the painting into sections: the observers are largely grouped under the left-hand window; Charcot is isolated between the small table with the scientific instruments and the right-hand window-shutter; the patient, 'Blanche', and the auxiliary medical staff are grouped under the right-hand window. Here, we are invited to look at the elements of the painting separately and consider their relationship to each other.

(9)   *Images of action*

The paintings by Rembrandt and Brouillet portray events, namely medical demonstrations. We can consider the nature of the action in such paintings: is it physical, mental or both? Who is acting on whom or what? How is the action portrayed? Are cultural groupings linked by the kind of actions they perform?

In Rembrandt's painting, Tulp displays an exposed part of the cadaver's arm with his right hand while his left hand makes the kind of gesture typical of a lecturer making a fine point: the forefinger and the thumb come together. His gaze, as noted above, is directed towards but above his audience, and certainly away from the cadaver. He is the teacher and his action is physical, on display. The observers, however, are engaged in learning: they gaze at the lecturer, the cadaver and steal a glance at the open textbook, the various sources of information. Their action is less visible, inferred from their various gazes. The cadaver, of course, plays no part in the action: it is inert, something to be stripped of flesh and exposed to public view.

In Brouillet's image, the clinician, Charcot, stands beside his patient but looks at his audience. Like Tulp, he makes a fine point by touching his forefinger to his thumb, but this time with his right hand. The other arm is by his side. The assembled male audience gazes at him and the patient, who leans back, her face towards the viewer, her eyes closed. The observers are in attitudes of attention: two support their heads with their hands, several have their heads to one side; several are taking notes. Again, the postures and actions of the observers suggest the mental activity of learning. By contrast, the three figures behind the patient are concerned only with her: they gaze at her with some apparent anxiety, and one holds her hands out as if ready to catch her. Here, the patient's role is ambiguous: she is alive but apparently unconscious. If the viewers know the story behind the painting, they will know that she is a hypnotised 'hysteric' and that Charcot's analysis and his methods of treatment were controversial, even in his own day. How much agency – if any? – does she have in the scene being portrayed? The viewer has to decide whether the patient is an active participant in the scene and whether or not she is 'performing' her symptoms for the doctor and his audience. Again, while portraying two apparently similar 'images of action', Rembrandt and Brouillet may be read as doing two rather different things: Rembrandt seeks to include his viewers in an educational event, meticulously detailed; Brouillet invites his viewer to consider what is actually happening in the episode and to reflect on the ethics of the relationship between lecturer, student and patient.

(10) *Descriptive images*

Often paintings or photographs do not show their elements in interaction; obviously, in medicine, part of the anatomy is often abstracted in a descriptive technical illustration that is intended to instruct the viewer, and, more generally, an individual might be portrayed for the viewer's contemplation and interpretation. Charcot, indeed, was a pioneer in the use of photography in medical illustration; he took photographs of patients adopting poses, hoping to identify gestures and expressions that were characteristic of hysteria. Many were published in *Nouvelle Iconographie de la Saltpêtrière* (1888). Viewers can therefore interrogate the cultural conventions governing descriptive images by asking questions about their purpose. Is the viewer expected to learn from what is portrayed, or is the image expected to evoke an emotional response such as desire, revulsion, fear, sympathy, curiosity or anger?

---

## Activity: Images of action and description

Find another image of a medical procedure and an image of a single individual, or part of an individual (e.g. by browsing the New York University Database at http://medhum.med.nyu.edu/).

(a) Describe the kind of setting, if any.

(b) Describe the composition of the image of action; how are the elements related to each other?

(c) How are the elements of the images framed? Are they shown as integrated wholes or as separated parts?

(d) In the action image, who is acting on whom or what? How is the viewer positioned in relation to the action?

(e) How is the viewer positioned in relation to the descriptive image? What kind of feeling – if any – is it expected to evoke?

# A Case Study: From Visual Analysis to Cultural Research

As we have shown above, images can be read as 'messages' and interpreted according to various cultural conventions that have developed over time. By attending to the questions suggested above, students can respond to images systematically and so develop routines that will enrich their visual literacy. However, images also enter into broader discourses, by accident or design, and these discourses can also stimulate discussion and debate in the medical education classroom. To illustrate how the 'message' embedded in an image can contribute to a wider cultural debate, we turn here to a painting of a famous episode in the history of medicine in Taiwan, an episode known as *A Loving Skin-graft* (see Figure 8.3). First we use the questions suggested in the foregoing section to interpret the painting; then, we look at ways of exploring the place of the painting in an enduring Taiwanese cultural myth (cf Landsborough, 1932, 1957; Wu, 2008).

In *A Loving Skin-graft*, the content includes a patient on his hospital bed, the doctors and nurses in attendance, a more shadowy figure in the

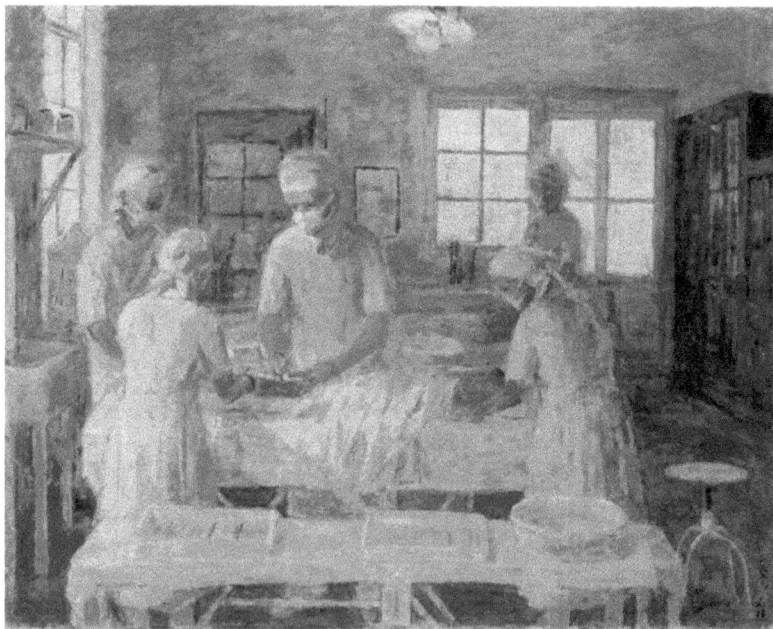

**Figure 8.3** *A Loving Skin-graft*, by Shi-Qiao Li

background, a table in the foreground on which are placed surgical instruments, the windows, cupboards and ceiling-light.

When considering content, we can reflect on the associations aroused by the figures on display. Medical figures, of course, and their instruments, may evoke respect or fear. Here the doctor and nurses are clothed in white and a bright light suffuses the room, suggesting cleanliness or tranquillity, possibly even spirituality. One of the nurses cradles the head of the patient in a compassionate manner. If we are aware that the patient is a young boy, then our sympathy for the vulnerable child might be accentuated. Unless the story behind the painting is known, the shadowy figure in the background may simply arouse curiosity, if she is noticed at all. It takes some scrutiny to notice that she is also lying on a bed, attended by another nurse.

This is a painting in which the important central space is occupied by the patient and medical staff. The shadowy female is removed slightly to the margin in the upper background to the right, framed by a window; and in the lower foreground there is a table with surgical instruments. The surgeon is placed at the centre of the medical staff; his is the only facial expression clearly visible to the viewer.

In *A Loving Skin-graft*, the surgeon's gaze is intently focused on the child's leg, which is being operated upon. Two of the other medical personnel also have their heads bowed, and they too are presumably looking at the leg. A nurse cradles the child's head and gazes at him, the obvious focus of her concern. No-one interacts directly with the viewer, who is positioned directly in front of the scene, which is, however, separated from the viewer by the table with the surgical instruments.

The viewer is thus invited to look upon this scene as if it is an isolated moment from a theatrical play or a film. Another possible, but more metaphorical, interpretation of the composition is that the viewer is situated before an altar table, on which surgical instruments are placed, and beyond the table some form of sacrifice is being made.

*A Loving Skin-graft* is not as realistic a painting as *The Anatomy Lesson of Dr Nicolaes Tulp* and medical students could not be expected to diagnose the patient's condition based on the sketchiness of his representation here. It is, rather, an impressionistic painting in style, dominated by the brilliant white of the medical staff's uniforms, the hospital bed and the low table of surgical instruments, which are pronounced against the relative darkness of the operating theatre. Although there are prominent windows and a light above, the radiance of the uniforms, bed and table is such that it may be interpreted symbolically: in western culture, white is the colour of purity and innocence, as well as the colour associated universally with cleanliness, and with scientific and medical clothing.

Some of the visual interpretation above is in part influenced by knowledge of the story that inspired it (Landsborough 1934, 1957; Wu, 2008): the doctor is David Landsborough, a Scottish medical missionary to Taiwan, who, in the late 19th century, began practising medicine in Changhua, where he founded a Christian hospital that opened in 1899. He married an English woman, Marjorie Leanner, in 1912, and in 1928 both were involved in the incident that gave rise to the painting. A 13-year-old boy, Kim Yao Chiu, grazed his knee on a rock; the wound became infected and the boy's stepfather treated the graze with traditional herbal remedies, which aggravated the infection. The father then took the child to visit a local practitioner of traditional medicine and a Taoist priest, but to no avail. By the time the child was brought to the Christian hospital in Changhua, the infection was so serious that the leg might have needed to have been amputated. Landsborough had read about but never practised the new art of skin-grafting; he considered this the best chance of saving the child's leg. Neither the child nor his stepfather was in a position to be a skin donor so Marjorie Landsborough agreed to donate skin from her own thigh in an attempt to heal Chiu. In the painting, Marjorie Landsborough is the shadowy figure lying in the background. The operation, however, was a failure, although once Chiu had regained more of his strength Landsborough did perform two further operations using some of Chiu's own skin, and after a year he was well enough to be discharged. By this time the child had become a close friend of Marjorie Landsborough, and, inspired by the sacrifice of her own skin by the medical missionary's wife, Chiu embraced the Christian faith and he himself became a Presbyterian pastor.

In the context of the story that inspired it, the painting can be seen as representing a moral and religious fable: a spiritual light suffuses the scene as the dedicated doctor and self-sacrificing wife labour to use new, western medical techniques to heal a boy whose condition has been worsened by a reliance on traditional herbal cures. The painting may be read as a celebration of Christian love, on the part of the donor, and the triumph of western medicine over traditional medicine and superstitious beliefs. As such, it is a painting that is – as Wu (2008) observed at a conference on Taiwanese Studies – ripe for revisitation.

Wu (2008) subjects the myth to critical scrutiny, comparing sources for the various versions of the tale. He observes that the episode celebrated by the painting has been transmitted in a variety of forms: Marjorie Landsborough mentioned it in her 1932 book of stories for children, but neglected to mention that she was the donor for the skin-graft operation, and she omitted the episode altogether from her brief 1957 biography of her husband. However, their son, David Landsborough IV, who was born in

Chunghua and who later worked there, affirmed that his mother was the donor to Dr Tsungming Tu, who visited Chunghua hospital in 1954. This oral testimony confirmed the story that Dr Tu had been told in 1941 by another physician, Dr Chen-Hui Su, who claimed to have assisted during the original operation. It was Dr Tu who then commissioned the painting from the artist Shi-Qiao Li (1908–1995). Dr Tu went on to found Kaohsiung Medical College, later Kaohsiung Medical University (KMU) in Taiwan, and Li's painting was hung in the foyer of KMU hospital, and the episode it illustrates was referred to explicitly in classes, in order to inspire succeeding generations of medical students. Indeed, a conference was held at KMU in 1998 to mark the 70th anniversary of the operation, and another painting of the episode, by Ying-yi Huang, was commissioned by the University in 2002.

Wu (2008) casts some doubt on the historical authenticity of the episode, noting that the original written hospital records were lost during World War II, and that the absence of factual data allowed the myth to evolve. He points out that David Landsborough II was a child in 1928, and attending boarding school some distance from Chuanghua, and that the other oral witness, Dr Chen-Hui Su, graduated in medicine two years after the operation took place, though he concedes that it is possible that Dr Su assisted Landsborough while still a medical student. What is certain is that the evidence of both men was transmitted by Tsungming Tu, who actively promoted the story of innovation and sacrifice to serve as the ethos of the medical college he founded. The operation shown in Li's painting can thus be interpreted as a miracle (although the operation had to be repeated twice); as a religious or secular parable of selfless sacrifice; and as a milestone in Taiwanese medical history. The story may thus be moulded to fit different purposes: it serves as Christian propaganda, as proof of the superiority of western biomedical practices and as evidence of Kaohsiung Medical University's affiliation with pioneering surgical techniques (though, as Wu also observes, KMU's claim in 1998 that Landsborough's skin-graft operation was a world first is clearly an exaggeration).

The painting, A Loving Skin-graft, then, can be seen as a document with a complex cultural history that resists unitary interpretation. Wu (2008: 16) argues that, in Taiwan, 'In medical schools, history is still taught by means of celebrating great works done by great figures.' In the intercultural language classroom, with medical students, Shi-Qiao Li's painting can be used alongside other narratives – for example, the published accounts of Marjorie Landsborough and Dr Tsungming Tu, and excerpts from Harry Yi-Jui Wu's conference paper – to explore the ways in which factual medical stories may be shaped and embellished to support and propagate different values, religious and secular.

---

### Activity: Outside the frame

Find a painting that has been used in medical education (e.g. by browsing the New York University Database at http://medhum.med.nyu. edu/).

(1) Find out as much as you can about its history – was it commissioned, who by, and where was it first displayed?
(2) Is the painting based on an actual event? If so, was the artist present or did he or she hear about it from another source or sources? How might the sources have interpreted the event? Did they have any agenda or propagandist purpose?
(3) Do you respond to the painting as a celebration or a criticism of the event being portrayed? What is the basis of your response – the style of the painting or your knowledge of the artist and his or her sources?
(4) Would a photograph of the event differ from the painting? Do different paintings of the same event exist? How would you describe the values represented by the event being portrayed?

---

## From Art as Image to Art as Concept and Practice

The use of the arts in medical education is now embedded in a number of medical curricula, though it takes, as we have seen, rather different forms in different places. Boisaubin and Winkler (2000: 292) suggest that 'Medical schools that do not have accessible fine arts or humanities programs may form allegiances with local artists to increase communication and understanding between these disciplines' and, indeed, in some medical schools, artists are invited to work directly with medical students. Lu (2010) interviewed the Scottish conceptual artist Christine Borland about her work in medical education. Borland's work includes 'Medicine Cabinet (Dessicated)' (2006), a set of framed, dried plants that correspond to those illustrated in a botanical work by Leonard Fuchs; and 'SimBodies, NoBodies' (2009) a grouping of plaster casts, medical mannequins and rubber moulds. Borland's involvement in the teaching of communication skills to medical students at Glasgow University gave rise to 'Simulated Patient' (2004) in which she examined observational skills, mirroring, empathetic listening, and body language in a series of interactive games and video installations that included recordings of medical students role-playing the delivery of bad news. Her work with students goes far beyond the development of visual literacy and the exploration of the cultural history of art works, as she outlined in her comments to Lu (2010: 94). They are worth quoting at length to illustrate the kinds of activity that artists and medical students can engage in together.

I'm sure that the good courses do much more than just give you a description of a painting. I've been involved with a medical school, the Peninsula Medical School in Cornwall, in Truro. They try to do much more than just the workshops and electives that I've been talking about, they actually are the only medical school in Britain, as far as I know, who have Medical Humanities at the core of the curriculum. It really doesn't feel tagged on. It feels as if thinking about things from an artist's perspective, or a writer's or a musician's, is built into every aspect. So, for example, if you're thinking about writing case notes, you're thinking about literature and the patient as a text. Artists are going along with medical students, and looking at patients and talking to patients in dermatology wards, for example, which is the classic situation where medical students look at the symptom. They may look at the rash without actually looking at the person. Whereas artists are, of course, looking at a bigger picture, and then they share experiences at the end of that, talking about what the artist has observed and what the medical student has observed. It seems like much more of an integrated way of looking and using the Humanities. I think some of the competences that you've indicated are very relevant and I think art can bring these things to medicine. What I'm trying to say is that that if the medical students are actually able to engage with thinking about making a piece of work, it can do a lot more than just the observation, whether they're observing a patient or a painting.

This kind of curricular innovation goes beyond the language classroom, but the types of competences it attempts to instil and the forms of reflective analysis of behaviour and values that are encouraged are evidently analogous to those addressed in intercultural language education. Where resources permit, then, there can be mutually fruitful interaction between practising artists and medical students, with the language or communication classroom acting as a potential interdisciplinary bridge.

## Moving Images: Film and Television

The concerns of this and the previous chapter come together in the use of film and television when teaching language and culture in medical education. Medical themes are popular in mainstream television drama, and they also abound in commercial and art-house cinema. Film and television presentations regularly combine striking visual images with a strong narrative that raises ethical and professional dilemmas. It is not surprising, then, that medical dramas are frequently used to raise ethical issues in medical educa-tion classes. Jobson and Knapp van Bogaert (2005) discuss the film *Lorenzo's Oil* (1992), commenting in detail on the tension between the conventions demanded by Hollywood drama and the complexities of the 'true story' on which the film is based. The film tells the story of two parents who strive to find a treatment for their son, Lorenzo's incurable disease, adrenoleukodystro-phy. The parents' efforts result in the use of an oil to treat the condition, and the treatment is followed by an improvement in Lorenzo's clinical condition. Jobson and Knapp van Bogaert conclude that while the film succeeds in its artistic intentions, it misrepresents the dates of the clinical trial of the treat-ment, it distorts the relationship between the parents' organisation and the health professionals involved for dramatic purposes, and it might ultimately be accused of raising false hopes in viewers who are suffering from the dis-ease, and their family and friends. In addressing the issues raised by the film, they suggest a series of questions to be asked of any fictional or fictionalised medical drama (Jobson & Knapp van Bogaert, 2005: 83–84); these have been slightly adapted as the basis of the activity below.

---

## Activity: Exloring ethics in medical drama

Watch a film or television programme that focuses on an ethical issue and be prepared to discuss the questions below:

(1)  Does the drama explore the complexities of the **ethical issue** fully, or does it exploit the issue for dramatic effect?
(2)  Discuss the portrayal of the **health workers** in the drama. Are they portrayed as compassionate professionals or not? Would you trust them? Is their role sentimentalised or made heroic? Are they por-trayed as fallible or as having greater powers over life and death than would normally be the case? How does the choice of actor or actress affect the viewer's response? How do factors such as lighting and camera angle affect the viewer's relation to the professionals?
(3)  Discuss the portrayal of the **patient** in the drama. Is the patient shown as having agency or as being passive? Is the portrayal ste-reotyped? How does the choice of actor or actress affect the

viewer's response? How do factors such as lighting and camera angle affect the viewer's relation to the patient?

(4)  Is the **disease or illness** portrayed one that is common and likely to be experienced by the average viewer or his or her family? Does the drama contribute to understanding of the condition or does it remain mysterious or frightening?

(5)  Does the drama address **alternative therapies**? If so, are they treated with sympathy or hostility? Is their portrayal in the drama justifiable?

(6)  Are medical **treatments** accurately portrayed in the drama? Are their side-effects portrayed in a balanced way? Are their benefits exaggerated?

(7)  Is the drama resolved with the patient's **cure**? If so, is this outcome sensationalised, as an apparent miracle, or is it shown in a reasonable context? Are the reasons for the cure made clear to the viewer? Does the cure rely on an important medical discovery; and, if so, are the circumstances surrounding the discovery simplified or over-dramatised?

(8)  Is the drama resolved with the patient's **death**? If so, is this death treated as the failure of the health system? Who or what is blamed? Or is death seen as a natural part of life?

(9)  If the drama relies on **comedy**, does this add or detract from the seriousness of many medical experiences? What is the nature of the comedy: is it farce or satire? Are the objects of satire individuals or institutions?

(10) Look at the **production** credits to see if technical advisers, experts or consultants have contributed to the drama. If so, are they medical professionals or those who have in some way experienced the illness (as patients or family)? Are there issues of confidentiality related to the drama? Is the publicity and marketing of the film ethically justifiable?

The questions posed provide a framework for addressing the many portrayals of health issues in film and on television. As with the use of single visual images, medical issues on film and on television can be treated in a 'classic' or 'avant garde' style. As Glasser (2005) observes, at one end of the cinematic spectrum is the mainstream Hollywood medical issue movie, such as *The Doctor* (1991), which, like *Lorenzo's Oil*, is 'based on a true story'. In this case the story is of a skilled but complacent surgeon, Jack McKee, who is diagnosed with throat cancer, and who is then compelled to view the system, of which he is part, from the defamiliarising perspective of the patient. At the other end of the spectrum is an art-house film like *Blue* (1993) in which the artist and director Derek Jarman has various artists narrate stories about AIDS over an unvarying blue background, for 80 minutes. Jarman was himself suffering from AIDS, and *Blue* was his final film. Boisaubin and Winkler (2000) include a discussion of popular or mainstream television and film in their outline of a possible medical humanities course, noting, for example, the shift in portrayals of fictional doctors on television from the young, romantic and idealised *Doctor Kildare* of the 1960s through the old and trustworthy *Marcus Welby M.D.* to the ethically more ambivalent (but still romanticised) characters who populate series like *House* and *Grey's Anatomy*. These American series have their British counterparts in programmes ranging from *Dr Finlay's Casebook* and *Emergency Ward 10* through to the long-running *Casualty*; antipodean medical series extend from *Emergency* in the 1950s to *All Saints*, which ended its run in 2009; and most other countries have similar series.

Popular medical dramas are, however, not without their critics in the medical profession. While aknowledging that two currently popular series, *House* and *Grey's Anatomy,* are designed to entertain rather than educate, Czarny *et al.* (2010: 205) demonstrate through a detailed content analysis of one season of each show that:

> television medical dramas are rife with depictions of bioethical issues and egregious deviations from the norms of professionalism. They contain exemplary depictions of professionalism to a much lesser degree.

For example, in the dramas sampled, the highest number of ethical dilemmas revolved around the issue of gaining patient consent (mainly in *House*); the norms of professionalism were most frequently breached in relation to sexual misconduct between professionals (mainly in *Grey's Anatomy*). The nature of the programmes can be related to these findings: *House* focuses on the work of Dr Gregory House, a brilliant but idiosyncratic physician in the mould of Sherlock Holmes (indeed, his name is a pun on 'House and Holmes'). The programmes focus on his deductive skill in puzzling out difficult cases, and in order to arrive at his brilliant conclusions he often resorts to unethical means. *Grey's Anatomy* dramatises the lives of five young surgical interns, and the basis of the stories is less to do with mysterious illnesses and more to do with evolving relationships. In the context of the programme, issues related to cultural competences can arise, if in a dramatically exaggerated way. In one episode from 2005 (Season 2, Episode 5: 'Bring the Pain'), an Asian patient and her father refuse to give consent to potentially life-saving heart surgery until a Hmong shaman has been brought to the hospital by helicopter to 'find her soul.' The issues of cultural misconceptions (even amongst well-meaning practitioners) that are raised by this episode are explored in greater depth in *The Spirit Catches You and You Fall Down* (Fadiman, 1998), a book about a Hmong child treated in the USA. The book raises a number of pertinent issues about culture, communication and the building of trust.

In their conclusions, Czarny *et al.* (2010: 206) caution that the complex and unresolved nature of many of the ethical issues portrayed in these medical dramas may be 'more likely to engage viewers in moral reflection than to shape their opinions in any particular direction'; in other words, the use of such dramas in medical education may have no predictable learning outcome. We noted in Chapter 7 our concurrence with Friedman (2002) that the teaching of ethics in medicine and addressing ethical dilemmas in the medical humanities must be seen as two distinctive sets of pedagogical practices: the latter is focused more on exploration of the medical students' own affective responses to medical situations, and a developing understanding of how medicine is situated in contemporary and historical cultures. Medical dramas can contribute to the latter set of pedagogical goals more than to the former. As discussed in Chapter 2, the invitation to engage in moral reflection with no guaranteed, specific outcome is one of Barnett's hallmarks of higher education: the student's values should be confronted, challenged and tested. However, Czarny *et al.*'s work reminds educators that simply exposing students to ethically challenging material through televised or filmed drama may not necessarily lead to the kind of learning processes that they desire. It is still necessary for teachers to provide a reflective framework for the students' viewing of visual images and medical dramas, if deeper learning is to be encouraged. Those engaged in intercultural language learning also need to support the learners' development of the communicative skills necessary to be able to discuss and critically evaluate visual, cinematic and televisual materials. These skills can be developed through the systematic use of visual materials, film and television in an educational context where similar questions – such as those suggested in the activities in this chapter – are asked about different images, films or programmes. In this way, students learn how to discover cultural information from visual materials, and they can reflect on the social and ethical values that are explored – or exploited – by these materials.

## Note

(1)  See, for example, the image and annotation at http://litmed.med.nyu.edu/Annotati on?action = view&annid = 12794

# 9 Course Design for Intercultural Language Education in Medical Settings

The previous chapters have outlined possible intercultural approaches to teaching English in medical education, from comparing the desired cultural competences of language students and medical students, and the means of teaching those competences, through the 'languastructure' and spoken genres of medical discourse, to critical cultural awareness through reflection on professional values, literature and art. Chapters 2–8 are intended to provide stimulation for readers to try out the approaches suggested; however, they do not in themselves constitute a course.

Naturally it is impossible to devise a single course that would suit the many contexts in which English is taught to medical students. The present chapter, then, covers some of the main considerations that constitute the process of language course design, and illustrates them with examples that are based on our own experience of intercultural language education in medical settings. The chapter covers the following areas (cf Nation & Macalister, 2010):

- principles of English for specific purposes;
- environment analysis;
- needs analysis;
- curricular goals;
- content and sequencing;
- format and presentation;
- monitoring and assessment;
- evaluation.

The chapter serves, then, not as a ready made course but as advice on how to draw upon the insights of the present volume when devising and adapting courses of your own.

# Principles of English for Specific Purposes

Teaching English in medical education, of course, qualifies as a mode of teaching English for specific purposes, or ESP (Belcher, 2009; Basturkmen, 2010). ESP developed in the 1960s, and is still driven by two powerful forces. The first is the claim by linguists that context-specific 'registers' and then 'genres' of language use could be comprehensively described. Register analysis, in brief, attempted to account for the characteristics of texts by relating them to three situational variables: the topic or domain of the text, the relationship between the producer and processor(s) of the text, and whether the text was written or spoken (e.g. Halliday *et al.*, 1964; Halliday & Hasan, 1985; Biber, 1988, 1995; Ghadessy, 1988). A medical case history, then, would fall into the domain of medicine, be directed by a clinician to fellow professionals with a high degree of knowledge about its content and conventions, and be characterised by features of narrative writing in summary form. Genre analysis developed from register analysis in different ways; one influential approach has been to account for textual features with reference to the purpose the text serves for the 'discourse community' that produced it (e.g. Swales, 1990; Bhatia, 1993; Hyland, 2000, 2006). The content and form of an oral medical case presentation would be related partly to two different purposes: first, to transfer information about a patient's condition, its cause and likely treatment, and second to demonstrate the junior doctor's knowledge and competence to senior colleagues. Together, the concepts of register and genre still underlie many linguistic characterisations of medical discourse (for different approaches, see Nwogu, 1997; Halkowski, 2011).

The second force driving ESP courses is that registers and genres can be related to the perceived 'needs' of adult second language learners in particular (e.g. Munby, 1978; West, 1994; Long, 2005). Needs analysis is predicated on the reasonable assumption that it is possible to predict, with some degree of certainty, some of the things that learners will be required to use the language for. Nevertheless, while the design of ESP courses around context-specific language and perceived learners' needs is still an established pedagogical procedure, it has to be granted that neither the concept of 'specific language' or 'specific needs' has developed unaltered over the past 50 years. The very notion of 'register' has undergone scrutiny, the latest formulation involving corpus-informed 'multi-dimensional analyses' that take into account the distribution of linguistic features across a number of situational factors, such as 'degree of involvement' (e.g. Conrad & Biber, 2001). In the 1990s, much scholarly energy shifted from register analysis towards a 'thicker' or 'ethnographic' analysis of genres, following Swales (1990), and even his working definition of linguistic varieties characterised by 'communicative purpose' has undergone various shifts in the last two decades, mostly in relation to the complex nature of the 'discourse communities' that share communicative purposes, and so share genres (e.g. Hyland, 2000, 2006).

Learners' 'needs' have proved no less elusive when scholars have attempted to define and categorise them. Munby's (1978) monograph on syllabus design launched a thousand post-graduate theses in Applied Linguistics, but later practitioners such as Hutchinson and Waters (1987) distinguish between learners' 'necessities' (what they need to perform their professional duties) and their 'wants' (what learners believe they need). The difference between these types of 'need' was brought home to one of the present authors early in his career when he devised a 'needs based' course for two Japanese scientists working for an international pharmaceuticals company, based on the knowledge that they would be required to present technical data in English at a conference in the UK. However, on meeting the workers, he discovered that their own priority was to learn the appropriate language to engage their English-speaking line manager in salary negotiations. Needs can be difficult to foresee. More recently, Benesch (1996: 724–5), following Robinson (1991) observed that the formulation of 'needs' is ideologically governed:

The lack of attention in needs analysis to sociopolitical issues and their effects on curriculum is due in part to the way social context is delineated in the EAP [English for Academic Purposes] literature. Social context is what takes place "outside our own classrooms" (Belcher & Braine, 1995, p. xiii) but not very far outside. It includes the discourse, classroom interactions, and assignments in courses across the disciplines but excludes the political and economic forces that influence life inside and outside academic institutions. Needs analysis has not considered social issues affecting students' current academic lives, such as ambivalence toward studying English or budget cuts, and those that may affect their future professional lives, such as deteriorating job opportunities. Yet students may need to examine these issues to understand the difficulties of pursuing a degree or getting a job or to participate in political processes that could improve their lives.

If the CEFR and American Standards curricular guidance (see Chapter 2) are understood as being governed by ideologically-conditioned 'needs', then these may be characterised as having an integrationist or acculturating agenda. The development of intercultural communicative competence is in part motivated by the wish for 'citizens of Europe' to be better equipped for the challenge of mutual comprehension of the plurality of European languages and cultures. The development of linguistic and cultural competence in the USA is driven more by the desire for immigrants to understand and accept the values governing their new environment, even as the members of the host community treat their home culture with equal understanding and respect. The adoption of the CEFR or American Standards outside their regions of origin is therefore ideologically problematical, though some aspects of the curricular guidance may indeed have a broader application.

When we move from more general to more specific 'needs' in medical settings, then the interplay between individual 'wants', institutional 'necessities' and social agendas is equally complex. A medical student may 'want' to study English for a number of personal reasons; these reasons will probably include becoming proficient enough in English to cope with the linguistic demands of the course content; they may or may not include learning to use English to reflect on professional values, to read literature or discuss art. The institution in which the student is studying medicine may demand that they learn through the medium of English, or at least read and write certain texts in English. For example, the current authors have been present at lectures on medicine that have been delivered in Chinese, but in which the accompanying slides and essential reading were in English. The institutional genres that the medical student needs to master may therefore vary from note taking in lectures, or reading textbooks and research, to participation in English language PBL scenarios (see Chapter 3). The focus of the present volume has, however, been largely on the social agenda: the community's desire that medical professionals adhere to an ethos that is realised through characteristics such as empathy, compassion and fairness. This social agenda is formulated, directly and indirectly, in institutional and external policy documents such as *Tomorrow's Doctors* (GMC, 1993, 2003, 2009), discussed in Chapter 2.

We recognise, with fellow language professionals, that course design is therefore a negotiation involving knowledge of the kind of language that learners are likely to need in order to function, first as students and then later as professional doctors, and knowledge of the personal, institutional and social 'needs' that the various stake-holders in medical education might or might not accept as relevant to their own situation. The following sections take up and extend some of the issues raised here, using Nation and

Mcalister's (2010) model of language curriculum design as a framework. Their model invites course designers to consider the environment in which teaching will occur, the needs of the learners, the goals of the curriculum, the sequencing of content, its format and presentation, how the students will be monitored and assessed, and how the course itself will be evaluated. We now take each of these topics in turn, illustrating them mainly with examples taken from our own experience of working with colleagues in Taiwan and the UK. However, the general principles can be extended to many other situations.

# Environment Analysis

An 'environment analysis' (Tessmer, 1990) involves a consideration of 'the nature of the learners, the teachers and the teaching situation' (Nation & Macalister, 2010: 2). Factors to consider here include:

- The learners' prior proficiency in English, their experience and maturity, their learning styles and their expectations of the English classes.
- The teachers' experience and training (especially with respect to intercultural language education and working with medical students).
- The amount of time available for English classes in the curriculum, the size of the classrooms, the teaching and learning resources available, and so on.

The course designer has more control over some of these issues than others. Given that an intercultural approach to teaching and learning English in medical settings is partly non-linguistic in nature, addressing as it does attitudes and values through self-reflection, both teachers and learners may initially be required to attend to written explanations of the rationale behind the course. If the rationale of the course is not accepted by students and teachers, then the course is unlikely to be successful. One way of addressing this issue is to turn it into a classroom activity, as below. Here, the activity is used with a class of Taiwanese medical students who take one year of English as part of a General Education programme, and another year of English for Medical Purposes, before progressing to pre-clinical training. Though generalisations are always to be treated with some scepticism, the Taiwanese Medical Accreditation Council (TMAC) notes on its website that compared with their international peers, Taiwanese students are relatively weak in reflection, the depth and breadth of their general knowledge, and maturity.[1] Though many have latent knowledge of English from high school, often they have had little practice in speaking and writing it, and lack confidence when communicating in real time. There is time, then, in the freshman and sophomore years of a General Education programme, to link students' interest in medicine with English courses that offer them the opportunity to broaden their general knowledge and develop their reflective skills alongside their language skills. Other students in other learning environments might have different constraints and therefore different priorities. However, whatever the learning environment, students and teachers should both be aware what the rationale for the course is, and the kinds of topic to be covered.

---

## Activity: Discussing the course rationale

In pairs, recall, if you can, an incident in which one of you visited a doctor because you were ill. What were the most important characteristics of the doctor? List them in order of importance:

(a) an excellent knowledge of medicine;
(b) a sympathetic manner;
(c) the ability to listen to your problems;
(d) experience of patients from different social backgrounds;
(e) the disposition to treat you fairly, without reference to your gender, race or social background.

Which of these characteristics do you think should be part of your medical education? How can courses in English contribute to these aspects of your medical education?

---

# Needs Analysis

As noted above, needs analysis has been the central plank of most ESP courses since the 1970s. Medical ESP, or English for Medical Purposes (EMP), of course, is itself a diverse area. Shi (2009) subdivides it into occupational EMP, for practising physicians and healthcare workers, and academic EMP, for medical students. Candlin et al. (1981) and Basturkman (2010: 88–107) offer detailed case studies of courses designed for practising medical doctors, focusing on the genre of doctor–patient consultation. There is nevertheless some blurring of the distinction between occupational and academic purposes, since senior medical students normally work as interns or clerks in hospitals, and so are also likely at some point to come into contact with patients and colleagues who use English as a first language or as a lingua franca or present with the support of an interpreter (cf Chapter 5). Even so, the immediate language needs that characterise each group will differ. If the medical degree is being delivered in English, the student will have a number of immediate academic needs (Shi, 2009: 206–7):

> For example, medical students, in order to successfully complete their education, need to master a large number of special medical terms in a short time (Lucas, Lenstrup, Prinz, Williamson, Yip & Tipoe, 1997), develop reading and listening skills (Chia, Johnson, Chia & Olive, 1999), practice active participation in class discussion, and improve writing skills for written examinations (Chur-Hansen, 1999, 2000).

Additionally, the various branches of academic medicine can be further divided into subject areas such as Dentistry, Nursing, Pharmacy, and so on, and the register and associated genres of each subject can be researched and treated appropriately. As we have seen, even if the subject is identical across educational institutions, the modes of teaching might range from traditional lecture to problem-based learning (Chapter 3).

As we have also seen above, needs themselves can be understood as *personal* (what the students want and recognise that they need), *institutional* (what the educational programme demands of the students) and *social* (what society through external validation bodies require of medical institutions and their students). Data about the different kinds of need can be gathered from student questionnaires (detailed examples are given in Chia *et al.*, 1999 and Huang & Lin, 2010), the analysis of student performance data (e.g. Shi *et al.*, 2001), as well as field observation and small-scale ethnographies of medical and academic settings (Shi, 2009: 215). What is less well represented in the literature is the examination of internal institutional policy statements and external documents such as the TACCT inventory (AAMC, 2006; see also Chapter 2).

To return to the case study mentioned at the end of the previous section, that is, the development of an intercultural medical English course for a group of freshman or sophomore students doing English as part of a General Education and EMP programme at a Taiwanese medical university, a needs analysis can draw upon published studies of comparable environments. Needs may change over time, as noted by Huang and Lin (2010) who revisit an analysis completed a decade earlier (Chia *et al.*, 1999), before the age of the internet and social media. Both studies used questionnaires to solicit the views of both students and teaching with regard to English language needs at a Taiwanese medical university comparable to the one discussed in the present case study. While Huang and Lin (2010: 49) found a high degree of interest in small-group teaching, and the use of television and film amongst medical students, the general conclusions of the earlier study were still borne out (Chia *et al.*, 1999: 115):

Students and faculty were in agreement that reading is the most important skill needed for students' medical studies, followed by listening, writing, and speaking, in that order, consistent with the findings of Guo (1987). Specifically, what students need is an understanding of textbooks and journal articles written in English, an understanding of lectures in which medical terms are given in English, and an ability to write reports and research papers. Further, students and faculty agreed on the problems students have with English in their medical studies, namely, limited vocabulary and slow reading speed, corroborating the findings of Guo (1987).

The students in our case study have roughly similar wants and needs: when interviewed they express an awareness of the importance of English to their studies, and they also express interest in using film and television in their language classes (cf. Chapter 8). What is missing from these studies is an awareness from all those questioned that English classes may contribute to medical education beyond the purely instrumental or pleasurable. In other words, in the outcomes, neither faculty nor students engage directly with the social agenda that we have argued may be addressed through language learning in medical settings. We suspect that this absence is a limitation of the needs analysis model as it has developed from Munby's (1978) 'narrow focus' on instrumental language (cf. Svendsen & Krebs, 1984; Nation & Macalister, 2010: 32); the very history of ESP teaching and learning, after all, has been characterised by an efficiency-driven impulse to abstract areas of professional experience from the broader humanistic concerns that have motivated the development of intercultural language education. Generally speaking, the critical exploration of social values has not been seen to be part of the remit of English for Business, or English for Science and Technology, for example. Nevertheless, there is no reason why ESP cannot address these values. An intercultural approach to English language teaching in medical settings is well-placed to extend the discourse of pedagogical needs beyond student 'wants' and 'institutional necessities' towards the abilities that are variously formulated as aspects of cross-cultural or intercultural communicative competence (Chapter 2).

Of course, this is not to say that student wants and institutional requirements are not important in course design. All three types of need must be addressed in a good course. In our case study of Taiwanese freshmen and sophomores, for example, we can satisfy the acknowledged interest in watching English-language television and films at the same time as introducing the affective, ethical and professional issues raised in Chapter 8. And, as noted in Chapter 3, we can address the institutional necessity of engaging in PBL scenarios in English and presenting case histories in English by preparing students through role-plays, discussions and project work that are also designed to develop intercultural communicative competence. The course designer's challenge is, within the environmental constraints of the institution, to devise a course that will address student wants, institutional necessities and the social agenda in ways that will be attractive to students and encourage them to enhance their language proficiency by actively engaging with the course content.

---

### Activity: Wants, Necessities and Social Agendas

Compare the needs analysis questionnaire that is included as an Appendix to Huang and Lin (2010) and the TACCT inventory of cross-cultural competences (AAMC, 2006).[2] How would you adapt the questionnaire for your students in the light of the TACCT inventory? In other words, can you devise a needs analysis questionnaire for your teaching environment that covers your student's perceived wants, your institutional necessities, *and* relevant aspects of cross-cultural competence?

---

# Curricular Goals

As with needs, the goals, aims or objectives of a curriculum have been and remain the subject of considerable debate. For example, within language education, curricular goals may be expressed in terms of:

• knowledge of language, for example, the learner's knowledge of general and technical vocabulary; ability to write a range of grammatically well-formed sentences;
• language skills, for example, the learner's ability to read, write, listen and speak in a range of contexts and at particular levels of proficiency;
• discursive competences, for example, the learner's ability to understand and operate in different discursive situations, such as doctor–patient consultations; consultations involving a mediator; oral or written examinations; case presentations to peers and superiors; and so on;
• intercultural *savoirs*/resources; for example, the learner's willingness to reflect critically on his or her own values; to demonstrate curiosity about the other; to identify ethnocentric perspectives; to draw on the poetic

resources of language; to mediate between conflicting interpretations of phenomena.

There are some who would argue that the expression of precise curricular objectives puts too great an emphasis on the desired products of education rather than the processes by which learners gain knowledge and skills (e.g. Hyland, 1997), and others who would wish to redirect attention away from, say, 'cultural competence' towards 'cultural humility' (Tervalon & Murray-Garcia, 1998). However, we follow Byram (1997: 56, 72n) in acknowledging the problematic issues involved in defining curricular goals or objectives, while maintaining the position that for reasons of 'comprehensiveness, coherence and transparency' it is useful for teachers and learners to understand the *intended* outcomes of any course, even if what is actually learned spills over from these intended outcomes, as it normally will.

An intercultural approach to teaching language and values in medical contexts will seek to address all the above goals. The course should give the students opportunity to use a range of language skills, and it should introduce students to the language of medicine, paying particular attention to technical and everyday expressions (Chapter 4). As we have seen, there is a now a wealth of guidance on coping with different discursive situations, like doctor-patient consultations and case presentations (Chapter 5). We suggest that the novel element in our course design, compared to many other EMP courses, is the introduction of intercultural communicative competence, but we have argued that this set of goals speaks directly to the social agenda and addresses issues of cross-cultural competence and shared decision making in the medical literature (Chapter 2).

---

### Activity: Reflecting on goals

Consider your own teaching environment, and your students' needs (including their personal wants, institutional necessities and social needs, as discussed above). What goals would you prioritise in your own medical English course?

- Language: medical vocabulary and grammar;
- Skills: reading, writing, speaking and listening to medically-related texts;
- Discourse: the conventional forms of interaction associated with particular medical settings;
- Intercultural goals: attitudes, values and beliefs.

# Content and Sequencing

Course designers' different assumptions about the consequences of progression dominate the pedagogical literature about the sequencing of course content. For example, Nation and Macalister (2010: 70–87) suggest that the units of progression in a course may be based on a successive exposure to particular grammatical realisations, or a phased engagement with the key vocabulary to be learned. The specification of the vocabulary may be based on frequency lists such as Coxhead's (2000) list of common academic vocabulary. However, Hyland and Tse (2007) raise questions about the usefulness of such 'general' lists, suggesting that discipline-specific lists should be generated for the students' own discipline; Gaviola (2002) discusses how this might be done using small corpora of medical articles (cf. Chapter 4). There is, however, a crucial problem in imagining the progression of a course as the step-by-step accumulation of linguistic items. Byram (1997: 75) expresses this problem eloquently:

> The images [of progression as climbing a ladder or making a journey] arise from ways of ordering the grammar of a language in pedagogically appropriate ways, some of which are intuitive or claim to be logical, others related to anticipated use of the language by learners, others derived from the order of learning by native speakers, and others appearing to arise from the structures of the language. Moreover, a pedagogical grammar may involve simplification of language structures in the early stages of learning, returning to present the full complexity at a later stage. In fact, it is only at the earlier stages of learning that the notion of each step depending on previous ones is evident. At later stages, the image of climbing a ladder can be replaced by the metaphor of completing a jigsaw puzzle, where the early stages have provided the edges and corners and at later stages learners, sometimes with the help of teachers, gradually complete elements of the whole picture without necessarily making connections among them until the picture is complete.

While course designers clearly need to be aware of the linguistic and intellectual complexity of the activities that learners are required to do, they do not necessarily need to be constrained by a linear model that gradually expands relevant vocabulary or grammatical realisations. In Chapter 2, we recommended a task-based syllabus as most relevant to language students in medical contexts, partly because a task-based approach is congruent with problem-based learning in medical education. Breen (2001: 155) observes that in task-based syllabuses, the course designer assumes that the learner 'refines knowledge and abilities in [a] cyclic way,' progressing from 'familiar to less familiar or generalisable to less generalisable tasks.' This accords with Byram's pleasing metaphor of the jigsaw puzzle; however, Nation and Macalister (2010: 81) are cautious about the ability of task-based to guarantee coverage of necessary language, arguing that:

> it is particularly important that there are other ways of checking the coverage of content, particularly vocabulary, grammar and types of discourse. Good curriculum design involves the checking of courses against a range of types of content.

In our case study, we suggest that the medical English course be organised around a series of topics. These may be more general or specific areas in medicine, depending on the students' own specialisations. Two possible sets of topics are shown in Table 9.1, based on two courses of different durations at Kaohsiung Medical University, one that covers medicine more generally, and the other that specialises in oral medicine:

**Table 9.1** Possible sequences of topic in a Medical English syllabus

| English for Medicine | English for Oral Medicine |
|---|---|
| 1. Mythology and medicine | 1. Gastrointestinal unit/cardiopathy unit |
| 2. Approach to medical terms and health professions | 2. Respiration unit |
| 3. Parts and functions of body | 3. Neurological unit |
| 4. Symptoms and signs, pronunciation | 4. Orthopedics unit |
| 5. Systems: Heart, circulation, and chest | 5. Urological unit |
| 6. Systems: Gastrointestinal, renal and endocrine | 6. Renal unit |
| 7. Gynaecology, pregnancy, childbirth | 7. Endocrine unit |
| 8. Childhood, infection, prevention | 8. Rectum unit |
| 9. Brain, mind and nervous system | 9. Infectious disease unit |
| 10. Taking a history and physical examination/ Investigations: Laboratory and image studies | 10. Oncology unit |
| 11. Global health | 11. Obstetrics unit |
| – | 12. Pediatrics unit |
| – | 13. Ear-nose-throat unit |
| – | 14. Ophthalmology unit |

These topics – or others like them – can provide the basis for a range of related language activities that cover key areas of intercultural communicative competence, as well as the vocabulary, grammar and discourse conventions associated with different medical settings. An example of one unit (English for Medicine 7: Gynaecology, pregnancy, childbirth) is given in the next section.

## Format and Presentation of Learning Materials

Different course designers will put together learning materials, resources and procedures that combine the general goals outlined above in a variety of ways. Nation and Mcalister (2010: 89–90) offer some general principles to guide the format and presentation of learning materials, a selection of which are summarised and adapted below:

(1)  The content of the course should be relevant and interesting to stimulate motivation.
(2)  The materials should include a balance of activities that focus on language (pronunciation, vocabulary, grammar and discourse structure) and focus on the exchange of meaning.
(3)  There should be exposure to interesting and accessible language in a range of reading and listening materials.
(4)  The learners should be encouraged to produce both written and spoken language fluently, over a range of discourse types.

In our Taiwanese case study, the curricular goals are embedded in topic-based units, such as 'Gynaecology, pregnancy and childbirth' (see previous section) which are clearly relevant to the students' clinical studies, and should therefore be motivational. The goals of this particular unit are addressed through a number of sample activities that employ four different types of input: (i) a news report on the CNN website about disparities in the provision of healthcare to pregnant women in impoverished countries around the world;[3] (ii) a UK National Health Service (NHS) website that instructs mothers-to-be on writing a 'birth plan' (see Chapter 6); (iii) an online corpus of general and technical language, the Corpus of Contemporary American English (see Chapter 4); (iv) the short story 'Hills like White Elephants' by Ernest Hemingway, first published in 1927, in which a young man attempts to persuade a young woman to have an abortion (Hemingway, 1966).

The topic of gynaecology, pregnancy and childbirth was introduced through the news, article, which introduced some key vocabulary and background knowledge on provision of healthcare across different cultures. Prompted by the NHS advice on writing a birth plan the students (male and female) were then asked to put themselves in the position of a pregnant mother and write and discuss their own preferred birth plans (see further, Chapter 6). Both the news story and the birth plan were then reviewed for vocabulary specifically related to gynaecology, pregnancy and childbirth; students explored this vocabulary further using the Corpus of Contemporary American English online, identifying academic and general uses of the words, and finding collocates and synonyms. Finally, the students read 'Hills Like White Elephants', which is in the form of a dialogue between a man and a woman whom he is trying to persuade to have an abortion (though this topic is never made explicit). The students need to use their inferencing skills to make explicit the topic of abortion; a post-reading activity might involve role-playing scenarios in which the man and/or the woman present at a clinic and request a termination. This scenario can lead to discussion of the values, ethics and official policies involved in terminations in different countries; in Taiwan, for example, consensus for abortion must be given by both the male and the female involved.

The distribution of activities and the goals they are intended to address are summarised in Table 9.2 below. This is, of course, only a sample of what might be done – the unit could be expanded into other areas, such as technical readings on aspects of gynaecology, or the materials suggested here could be adapted in different ways. For example, the short story could be used in a more formal way as part of a PBL 'trigger' as in Chapter 3; or the students might be asked to discuss visual representations of childbirth, such as Frida Khalo's 'Frida and the Miscarriage' or Alice Neel's 'Well Baby Clinic' using the techniques outlined in Chapter 8. Our point here is simply to demonstrate possible ways of formatting and presenting materials that address different kinds of curricular goals.

---

### Activity: Analysing your own course materials

Consider a medical English textbook that you use, or some materials you have designed to teach English to medical students. Which of the various possible goals discussed above – *linguistic, skills-based, discursive, intercultural* – do the textbook/materials address? How might you adapt the materials to address a wider range of curricular goals?

**Table 9.2** Distribution of goals in a sample unit on 'Gynaecology, Pregnancy and Childbirth'

| Goals | | | | | |
|---|---|---|---|---|---|
| Linguistic | Skills-based | Discursive | Intercultural | Input | Activity |
| Medical vocabulary (general) | Scanning for information (reading) | Reading a general news article | Comparing facts across cultures | News article | Reading for information |
| Medical vocabulary (general) | Writing from a particular perspective | Writing a birth plan | Empathy with mothers-to-be | NHS birth plan | Writing and discussion |
| Medical vocabulary (general and technical) | Skimming and scanning (reading) | Using language reference tools | Comparing professional and non-professional terminologies | Online corpus | Search for frequency, collocations and synonyms |
| Medical vocabulary | Reading in depth (inferencing); speaking | Reading a literary text; role-playing doctor-patient consultation | Empathy with characters in story: exploring values through role-play and discussion | Short story: 'Hills Like White Elephants' | Reading and inferencing; role-play and discussion |

# Monitoring and Assessment

The research literature on language assessment is, of course, vast. The role that language assessment plays in the progress of students through medical courses will vary considerably: language assessment may be integrated into some medical courses, in some ways, or the language programme may be an unassessed adjunct to the medical degree. Here, then, we can give only relatively general advice on why and how students' developing intercultural communicative competence may be assessed. This, in itself, is a complex area, which is addressed in detail in Byram (1997); some further practical advice is given also in Lázár et al. (2007).

There are, of course, good arguments for the assessment of students, even when it is not a formal requirement, and these are well rehearsed in the literature, from detailed discussions such as are found in Clapham and Corson (1997) to overviews such as Brindley (2001). Students may be assessed to place them on a course at an appropriate level; to diagnose their abilities and their needs, usually in relation to institutional necessities; to gauge how they are progressing through a course (formative assessment); and to determine their level of achievement when the course has ended (summative assessment). Language tests can take the form of discrete item objective tests (e.g. multiple-choice vocabulary tests, which can be automatically marked), or subjective assessment can take the form of freer composition or less controlled spoken interactions.

Standardised language tests are not the ideal means of assessing the development of intercultural communicative competence, and preferred means of assessment instrument might include structured observation of performance in particular scenarios (e.g. case presentations, or PBL), learning journals, project work, peer-assessment and self-assessment (cf. Brindley, 2001: 142). Byram (1997) suggests using a range of data in 'portfolios' to gather evidence for intercultural communicative competence; the European Language Portfolio (e.g. Little, 2002) gives further illustration of the range of the use of potential learning instruments such as the 'language biography' (cf. also Byram et al., 2009). While many of these learning and assessment instruments have not been designed specifically for medical students, they may be adapted for use in medical settings. Byram et al.'s (2009) 'Autobiography of Intercultural Encounters', for example, can be adapted specifically for medical encounters. Adapted excerpts are given in Figure 9.1 as possible prompts for reflective writing. This kind of reflection can also be done in relation to video recordings of interactions between doctors and patients of different cultural backgrounds (e.g. Moss & Roberts, 2003; Roberts et al., 2008).

An intercultural doctor-patient consultation can be a consultation that with someone from a different country, but it can also be a consultation with someone from another cultural background in your country. It might be, for example, a consultation with a patient from another region, someone who speaks a different language, someone from a different religion or from a different ethnic group.

This focus is on ONE patient consultation which you have had with someone different from yourself. It may be a new patient, or somebody you already know and have known for some time.

*** 

Imagine yourself in the patient's position...
*How do you think the patient felt in the situation at the time? This can be difficult but try and imagine what they felt at the time. Happy or upset/stressed, or what? How did you know?*
*What do you think they were thinking during the consultation? Do you think they found it strange, or upsetting, or reassuring, or what?*
Choose one or more of these or add your own and say why you have chosen it.
For them it was an unusual consultation / a surprising consultation / a shocking consultation / because...

**Figure 9.1** Adaptation of 'Autobiography of Intercultural Encounters' (Byram *et al.*, 2009)

As well as autobiographical and reflective writing, students may be asked to perform particular speaking tasks – for example, they may be required to take a particular role in a PBL scenario – and criteria for assessment can be applied to their performance (cf. the PBL assessment schemes devised by Valle *et al.*, 1999 and Sim *et al.*, 2006). Sim *et al.* (2006: 636) for example, present a simple and useful coding scheme used at the University of Malaya, which scores students' performance in PBLs across a range of criteria, such as:

- participation and communication skills;
- cooperation/team-building skills;
- comprehension/reasoning skills;
- knowledge/information-gathering skills.

Students may also be trained to self-assess their performance in such contexts (but see Eva, 2001 for reflections on the challenges of taking this option).

The main goal of assessment here is clearly to promote learning. Assessment that relates closely to the course goals and addresses the students' perceived needs can have a motivational benefit in that it legitimises the learning activities of the course and demonstrates tangible progress. Assessment also helps give the teacher and course designers feedback that is valuable when planning future versions of the course; however, this is a topic that properly belongs to the following section.

# Evaluation

Wall (2010) provides a succinct overview of issues to address when evaluating courses in medical education. Course evaluation may overlap with student assessment in some details; however, its purpose is and should be kept distinct. Those involved in running courses evaluate them to monitor a number of factors that contribute to the overall quality of the course, for example,

- the quality of the teaching;
- student satisfaction;
- whether stated course outcomes were delivered;
- availability of learning resources, support, and so on.

The nature and depth of the evaluation will depend in part on its audience; for instance, is the evaluation teacher-directed as part of on-going professional development, or is it part of an external evaluation of the quality of provision at your institution? This information will feed into the initial stage of what will then become an on-going cycle of evaluation as expressed by Genesee (2001: 145):

(1)  Articulate the purposes of the evaluation.
(2)  Identify and collect data.
(3)  Analyse and interpret the data.
(4)  Make decisions about changes to the course.

The sources of data for evaluation are various. They may come from talking to the teaching staff and students, formally or informally; analysing the outcomes of student assessments; reviewing the responses to particular course materials; reading the minutes of department meetings; and so on (cf Nation & Macalister, 2010: 128–133). More broadly, evaluation can be informed by attendance at educational conferences; visits to institutions delivering similar courses; undertaking graduate research in a relevant discipline; reading the pedagogical and research literature. As with most areas of education, evaluation is a complex issue, loaded with its own ideological freight, given that management, teachers and students often have divergent interests when they consider whether a particular course is successful or unsuccessful.

# Conclusion

The roots of the present volume lie in the authors' interest in intercultural language education generally, and the specific challenges of implementing an intercultural approach to language teaching in the context of an English programme in a medical university (Corbett, 2003; Lu, 2006). Our thinking was then profoundly affected by attending a conference on 'Cultural Competence in Medical Education' held at Kaohsiung Medical University in 2008, where we both had the opportunity to engage with experts in cross-cultural competence in medical education and training; we had also begun to explore ways of using digital resources in our teaching, and to consider the role that the medical humanities might play in an intercultural approach to teaching English in medical settings. The present volume, then, is our attempt to make sense of and intervene in a fast-changing educational field. The preceding chapters set out to explain the parallels between intercultural communicative competence and cultural competence in medical education; to identify cognate means of task and problem-based learning in language and medicine; to suggest ways of exploring medical language and of understanding medical talk; and to encourage critical cultural awareness through reflection on professional values and engagements with literature and art. The present chapter sought to illustrate how the issues raised in the preceding chapters might be applied in the design of English courses for medical students. No doubt the field will continue to develop, but we hope that readers find this a useful contribution to an on-going dialogue between language and medical education.

## Notes

(1) http://www.heeact.edu.tw/lp.asp?ctNode = 340&CtUnit = 108&BaseDSD = 7& mp = 3
(2) Both documents are available online: Huang and Lin (2010) at www.asian-esp-journal.com/May_2010_Ebook.pdf and AAMC (2006) at www.aamc.org/meded/tacct/tacctresourceguide.pdf
(3) The case study used the article 'When joy of pregnancy turns to heartbreak' (2009) retrieved from http://articles.cnn.com/2009-01-22/world/veneman.childbirth_1_sierra-leone-prenatal-care-child-mortality-rates?_s = PM:WORLD. However, as health disparities in childcare is a common topic in news reporting, the article may be substituted by an more up-to-date one.

# References

Adolphs, S., Brown, B., Carter, R., Crawford, P. and Sahota, O. (2004) Applied clinical linguistics: Corpus linguistics in health care settings. *Journal of Applied Linguistics* 1, 9–28.

Aijmer, K. (ed.) (2009) *Corpora in Language Teaching*. Amsterdam: John Benjamins.

Agar, M. (1994) *Language Shock: Understanding the Culture of Conversation*. New York:
William Morrow.

Albanese, M.A. (2010) Problem-based learning. In T. Swanwick (ed.) *Understanding Medical
Education: Evidence, Theory and Practice* (pp. 37–52). Oxford: Wiley-Blackwell.

Allum, V. and McGarr, P. (2010) *Cambridge English for Nursing: Pre-Intermediate*. Cambridge:
Cambridge University Press.

American Council for the Teaching of Foreign Languages [ACTFL] (1996) *Standards for
Foreign Language Education: Preparing for the 21st Century*. Alexandria, VA: ACTFL, Inc.

Americano, A. and Bhugra, D. (2010) Dealing with diversity. In T. Swanwick (ed.)
*Understanding Medical Education: Evidence, Theory and Practice* (pp. 392–402). Oxford:
Wiley-Blackwell.

Anderson, J., Barnes, E. and Shackleton, E. (2011) *The Art of Medicine: Over 2000 Years of
Medicine in Our Lives*. Lewes: Ilex Press and the Wellcome Collection.

Anderson, T., Howe, C., Soden, R., Haliday, J. and Low, J. (2001) Peer interaction and the
learning of critical thinking skills in further education students. *Instructional Design*
29, 1–32.

Anderson, W. and Corbett, J. (2009) *Exploring English with Online Corpora*. London:
Palgrave Macmillan.

Angell, M. and Kassirer, J.P. (1998) Alternative medicine – the risks of untested and unreg-
ulated remedies. *New England Journal of Medicine* 339, 839–841.

Anspach, R.R. (1988) Notes on the sociology of medical discourse: The language of case
presentation. *Journal of Health and Social Behavior* 29 (4), 357–375.

Anthony, D. (2009) Low-tech solution to a high-tech problem. *Virtual Mentor* 11 (3), 202–
206. [Retrieved from http://virtualmentor.ama-assn.org/2009/03/ccas1-0903.html].

Association of American Medical Colleges [AAMC] (2005) *Cultural Competence Education
for Medical Students*. Washington, DC: AAMC. [Retrieved from https://www.aamc.
org/download/54338/data/culturalcomped.pdf]

Association of American Medical Colleges [AAMC] (2006) *TACCT Resource Guide*.
Washington, DC: AAMC. [Retrieved from http://www.aamc.org/meded/tacct/
tacctresourceguide.pdf]

Atkinson, D. (1992) The evolution of medical research writing from 1735 to 1985: The
case of the *Edinburgh Medical Journal*. *Applied Linguistics* 13 (4), 337–374.

Bailey, B. (2000) Communicative behaviour and conflict between African-American customers and Korean immigrant retailers in Los Angeles. *Discourse and Society* 11 (1), 87–108.

Balshem, M. (1991) Cancer, control, and causality: Talking about cancer in a working-class community. *American Ethnologist* 18 (1), 152–172.

Baker, P. (2006) *Using Corpora in Discourse Analysis*. London and New York: Continuum.

Bamforth, I. (ed.) (2003) *The Body in the Library: A Literary History of Modern Medicine*. London and New York: Verso.

Baraldi, C. (2009) Forms of mediation: the case of interpreter-mediated interactions in medical systems. *Language and Intercultural Communication* 9 (2), 120–137.

Barker, K. (1998) A ship upon a stormy sea: The medicalization of pregnancy. *Social Science and Medicine* 47 (8), 867–884.

Barone, A.D., Yoels, W.C. and Clair, J.M. (1999) How physicians view caregivers: Simmel in the examination room. *Sociological Perspectives* 42 (4), 673–690.

Barnett, R. (1994) *The Limits of Competence: Knowledge, Higher Education and Society*. Buckingham: Open University Press.

Barrows, H.S. (1996) Problem-based learning in medicine and beyond: A brief overview. *New Directions for Teaching and Learning* 68, 3–12.

Basturkmen, H. (2010) *Developing Courses in English for Specific Purposes*. London: Palgrave Macmillan.

Bauby, J-D. (1997) *The Diving-Bell and the Butterfly*, trans. J. Leggatt. New York: Alfred A. Knopf.

Beckett, S. (1983) *Worstward Ho*. London: John Calder.

Beitler, L. and Macdonald, B. (1982) *English for the Medical Professions*. New York: McGraw-Hill.

Belcher, D. (2009) Problem-solving for nursing purposes. In D. Belcher (ed.) (2009) *English for Specific Purposes in Theory and Practice* (pp. 229–242). Ann Arbor: University of Michigan Press.

Belcher, D. (ed.) (2009) *English for Specific Purposes in Theory and Practice*. Ann Arbor: University of Michigan Press.

Belcher, D. and Braine, G. (eds) (1995) *Academic writing in a second language: Essays on Research and Pedagogy*. Norwood NJ: Ablex.

Belz, J. A. (2003) Linguistic perspectives on the development of intercultural competence in telecollaboration. *Language Learning and Technology* 7 (2), 68–99.

Benesch, S. (1996) Needs analysis and curriculum development in EAP: An example of a critical approach. *TESOL Quarterly* 30 (4), 723–738.

Bennett, G. (2010) *Using Corpora in the Language Learning Classroom*. Ann Arbor: University of Michigan Press.

Benson, P. (2002) Rethinking the relationship of self-access and autonomy. *Self-Access Language Learning* 5 (Newsletter of the Hong Kong Association for Self-Access Learning and Development), 4–10.

Berger, J. and Mohr, J. (1967) *A Fortunate Man: The Story of a Country Doctor*. Harmondsworth: Penguin.

Betancourt, J.R. (2003) Cross-cultural medical education: Conceptual approaches and frameworks for evaluation. *Academic Medicine* 78 (6), 560–569.

Betancourt, J.R. (2004) Cultural competence – marginal or mainstream movement? *The New England Journal of Medicine* 351 (10), 953–955.

Betancourt, J.R. (2006) Cultural competency: Providing quality care to diverse populations. *The Consultant Pharmacist* 21 (12), 988–995.

Betancourt, J.R., Green, A.R., Carrillo, J.E. and Ananeh-Firempong II, O. (2003) Defining cultural competence: A practical framework for addressing racial/ethnic disparities in health and health care. *Public Health Reports* 118, 293–302.

Bhatia, V.K. (1993) *Analysing Genre: Language Use in Professional Settings*. Harlow: Longman.

Biber, D. (1988) *Variation across Speech and Writing*. Cambridge: Cambridge University Press.

Biber, D. (1995) *Dimesions of Register Variation: A Cross-linguistic Comparison*. Cambridge: Cambridge University Press.

Biber, D. and Finegan, E. (1994) Intra-textual variation within medical research articles. In N. Oostdijk and P. de Haan (eds) *Corpus-Based Research into Language* (pp. 201–222). Amsterdam: Rodopi.

Bloom, G. (1982) *The Language of Medicine in English*. Englewood Cliffs, N.J.: Prentice Hall.

Boisaubin, E.V. and Winkler, M.G. (2000) Seeing patients and life contexts: The visual arts in medical education. *American Journal of Medical Sciences* 319 (5), 292–296.

Bok, D. (2006) *Our Underachieving Colleges: A Candid Look at How Much Students Learn and Why They Should Be Learning More*. New Jersey: Princeton University Press.

Bondi, M., Gavioli, L. and Silver, M. (eds) (2004) *Academic Discourse, Genre and Small Corpora*. Rome: Officina Edizioni.

Borland, C. (2004) *Simulated Patient*. Exhibited at the Lisson Gallery, London. [ http://www.studio55.org.uk/researchers/christine/simulated.html#nogo]

Bourdieu, P. (1979) *La Distinction Critique Social du Judgement*. Paris: Editions du Minuit.

Bourdieu, P. (1984) *Distinction: A Social Critique of the Judgement of Taste*, trans. R. Nice. Cambridge, MA: Harvard University Press.

Boyle, J.P. (1986) Testing language with students of Literature in ESL situations. In C.J. Brumfit and R.A. Carter (eds) *Literature and Language Teaching* (pp. 199–207). Oxford: Oxford University Press.

Breen, M.P. (2001) Syllabus design. In R. Carter and D. Nunan (eds) *The Cambridge Guide to Teaching English to Speakers of Other Languages* (pp. 151–159). Cambridge: Cambridge University Press.

Brindley, G. (2001) Assessment. In R. Carter and D. Nunan (eds) (2001) *The Cambridge Guide to Teaching English to Speakers of Other Languages* (pp. 137–143). Cambridge: Cambridge University Press.

Brown, B.J., Crawford, P. and Carter, R. (2006) *Evidence-Based Health Communication*. Maidenhead: McGraw-Hill/Open University Press.

Brown, B.J., Harvey, K.J., Churchill, R., Crawford, P., Mullany, L., McFarlane, A. and McPherson, A. (2008) Health communication and adolescents: What do their emails tell us? *Family Practice* 25, 304–311.

Burbaum, C., Stresing, A-M., Fritzsche, K., Auer, P., Wirsching, M. and Lucius-Hoene, G. (2010) Medically unexplained symptoms as a threat to patients' identity? A conversation analysis of patients' reactions to psychosomatic attributions. *Patient Education and Counseling* 79, 207–217.

Byram, M. (1997) *Teaching and Assessing Intercultural Communicative Competence*. Clevedon: Multilingual Matters.

Byram, M. (2008) *From Foreign Language Learning to Learning for Intercultural Citizenship: Essays and Reflections*. Clevedon: Multilingual Matters.

Byram, M., Barrett, M., Ipgrave, J., Jackson, R. and García, M.C.M. (2009) *Autobiography of Intercultural Encounters*. Strasbourg: Council of Europe [Retrieved from http://www.coe.int/t/dg4/autobiography/Source/AIE_en/AIE_autobiography_en.pdf].

Byram, M., Zarate, G. and Neuner, G. (1997) *Sociocultural Competence in Language Learning and Teaching*. Strasbourg: Council of Europe.

Byram, M. and Fleming, M. (eds) (1998) *Language Learning in Intercultural Perspective: Approaches through Drama and Ethnography.* Cambridge: Cambridge University Press.

Byrnes, H. (2006) Locating the advanced learner in theory, research and educational practice: An introduction. In H. Byrnes, H. Weger-Guntharp and K.A. Sprang (eds) *Educating for Advanced Foreign Language Capacities: Constructs, Curriculum, Instruction, Assessment* (pp. 1–14). Washington, DC: Georgetown University Press.

California Endowment (n.d.) *Connecting Worlds: Training for Health Care Interpreters.* Manual and Workbook. Los Angeles: California Endowment. [Retrieved from http://www.calendow.org/uploadedFiles/connecting_worlds_manual.pdf and http://www.calendow.org/uploadedFiles/connecting_worlds_workbook.pdf]

California Healthcare Interpreters' Association (2002) *California Standards for Healthcare Interpreters: Ethical Principles, Protocols, and Guidance on Roles and Intervention.* Los Angeles: California Endowment. [Retrieved from http://www.interpreterschia.org/standards/standards_home.htm.]

Calman, K.C. (1997) Literature in the education of the doctor. *Lancet* 350, 1622–1624.

Cameron, R. and Williams, J. (1997) Senténce to ten Cents: A case study of relevance and communicative success in nonnative-native speaker interaction in a medical setting. *Applied Linguistics* 18 (4), 415–445.

Campinha-Bacote, J. (1999) A model and instrument for assessing cultural competence in health care. *Journal of Nursing Education* 38 (5), 203–207.

Canale, M. and Swain, M. (1980) Theoretical bases of communicative approaches to second language teaching and testing. *Applied Linguistics* 1, 1–47.

Candlin, C.N., Bruton, C.J., Leather, J.H. and Woods, E.G. (1981) Designing modular materials for communicative language learning; an example: Doctor-patient communication skills. In L. Selinker, E. Tarone and V. Hanzeli (eds) *English for Academic and Technical Purposes: Studies in Honour of Louis Trimble* (pp. 105–133). Rowley MA: Newbury House.

Candlin, C.N. and Candlin, S. (2003) Health care communication: A problematic site for applied linguistics research. *Annual Review of Applied Linguistics* 23, 134–154.

Carter, R. and Long, M.N. (1995) *Teaching Literature.* London: Longman.

Carter, R. and Nunan, D. (eds) (2001) *The Cambridge Guide to Teaching English to Speakers of Other Languages.* Cambridge: Cambridge University Press.

Carter, Y.H., Skelton, J.R., Kenkre, J.E. and Hobbs, F.D.R. (1997) Analysis of primary care staff language about aggression at work using concordancing techniques to identify themes. *Family Practice* 14 (2), 136–141.

Chan, L.K. and Shum, M.K.S. (2011) Analysis of Students' Reflective Essays on Their First Human Dissection Experience. *Korean Journal of Medical Education* 23 (3), 209–219.

Chen, Cheng-Sheng, Chung-Sheng Lai, Peih-Ying Lu, Jer-Chia Tsai, Hung-Che Chiang, In-Ting Huang and Hsin-Su Yu. (2008) Performance anxiety at English PBL groups among Taiwanese medical students: A preliminary study. *The Kaohsiung Journal of Medical Sciences* 24 (3), Supplement 1, S54–S58.

Charon, R. (2000) Literary concepts for medical readers: Frame, time, plot, desire. In A.H. Hawkins and M.C. McEntyre (eds) *Teaching Literature and Medicine* (pp. 29–41). New York: Modern Languages Association of America.

Charon, R. (2005) Narrative medicine: Attention, representation, affiliation. *Narrative* 13 (3), 261–270.

Charon, R. (2006) *Narrative Medicine: Honoring the Stories of Illness.* New York: Oxford University Press.

Charon, R. (2007) What to do with stories: The sciences of narrative medicine. *Canadian Family Physician/Le Médecin de famille canadien* 53, 1265–1267.

Cheng, W. and Warren, M. (2006) //you need to be RUTHless//: Entertaining cross-cultural differences. *Language and Intercultural Communication* 6 (1), 35–56.

Chia, H-U., Johnson, R., Chia, H-L. and Olive, F. (1999) English for college students in Taiwan: A study of perceptions of English needs in a medical context. *English for Specific Purposes* 18 (2), 107–119.

Chomsky, N. (1965) *Aspects of the Theory of Syntax*. Cambridge, MA: MIT Press.

Chur-Hansen, A. (1999) Teaching support in the behavioural sciences for non-English speaking background medical undergraduates. *Medical Education* 33 (6), 404–410.

Chur-Hansen, A. (2000) Medical students' essay-writing skills: Criteria-based self- and tutor-evaluation and the role of language background. *Medical Education* 34 (3), 194–198.

Clair, J.M. (1990) Regressive intervention: The discourse of medicine during terminal encounters. *Advances in Medical Sociology* 1, 57–97.

Clapham, C. and Corson, D. (eds) (1997) *Language Testing and Assessment, Encyclopedia of Language and Education*. Vol. 7. Dordrecht: Kluwer.

Clare, A. (1991) Developing communication and interviewing skills. In R. Corney (ed.) *Developing Communication and Counselling Skills in Medicine* (pp. 16–24). London and New York: Tavistock/Routledge.

Clark, J.L. (1987) Classroom assessment in a communicative approach. *British Journal of Language Teaching* 25 (1), 9–19.

Cohn, S.K. (2010) *Cultures of Plague: Medical Thinking at the End of the Renaissance*. Oxford: Oxford University Press.

Coles, R. (ed.) (1984) *The Doctor Stories*. New York: New Directions.

Collett, T. and McLachlan, J.C. (2006) Evaluating a poetry workshop in medical education. *Medical Humanities* 32 (1), 59–64.

Conrad, S. and Biber, D. (eds) (2001) *Variation in English: Multidimensional Studies*. Harlow: Longman.

Coombs, R.H. and Goldman, L.J. (1973) Maintenance and discontinuity of coping mechanisms in an intensive care unit. *Social Problems* 20, 342–355.

Corbett, J. (2003) *An Intercultural Approach to English Language Teaching*. Clevedon: Multilingual Matters.

Corbett, J. (2010) *Intercultural Language Activities*. Cambridge Handbooks for Language Teachers. Cambridge: Cambridge University Press.

Corbett, J. (2011) Discourse and intercultural communication. In K. Hyland and B. Paltridge (eds) *The Continuum Companion to Discourse Analysis* (pp. 306–320). London and New York: Continuum.

Corney, R. (ed.) (1991) *Developing Communication and Counselling Skills in Medicine*. London and New York: Tavistock/Routledge.

Council of Europe (2001) *Common European Framework of Reference for Languages: Learning, Teaching, Assessment*. Cambridge: Cambridge University Press.

Coxhead, A. (2000) A new academic word list. *TESOL Quarterly* 34 (2), 213–238.

Crawford, P. and Brown, B.J. (2010) Health communication: Corpus linguistics, data driven learning and education for health professionals. *International English for Specific Purposes Journal* 2, 1–26.

Cronin, A.J. (1937) *The Citadel*. Boston: Little, Brown and Co.

Cross, T., Bazron, B., Dennis, K. and Isaacs, M. (1989) *Towards a culturally competent system of care Vol. 1*, National Technical Assistance Center for Childrens Mental Health, Georgetown University Child Development Center, Washington DC and NWICWA;

see also http://gucchd.georgetown.edu/programs/ta_center/topics/cultural_linguistic_competence.htm)

Czarny, M.J., Faden, R.R. and Sugarman, J. (2010) Bioethics and professionalism in popular television medical dramas. *Journal of Medical Ethics* 36 (4), 203–206.

Damen, L. (1987) *Culture Learning: The Fifth Dimension in the Language Classroom*. Boston: Addison-Wesley.

Dammers, J., Spencer, J. and Thomas, M. (2001) Using real patients in problem-based learning: students comments on the value of using real, as opposed to paper cases, in a problem-based learning module in general practice. *Medical Education* 35, 27–34.

David, T., Patel, L., Burdett, K. and Rangachari, P. (1999) *Problem-based Learning in Medicine*. London: Royal Society of Medicine.

Davidhizar, R., Giger, J.N. and Hannenpluf, L.W. (2006) Using the Giger–Davidhizar transcultural assessment model (GDTAM) in providing patient care. *The Journal of Practical Nursing* 56, 20–25.

De Jong, W. (1996) *Open Frontiers: Teaching English in an Intercultural Context*. Oxford: Heinemann.

Diemers, A.D., Dolmans, D.H., Van Santen, M., Van Luijk, S.J., Janssen-Noordman, A.M. and Scherpbier, A.J. (2007) Students perceptions of early patient encounters in a PBL curriculum: A first evaluation of the Maastricht experience. *Medical Teacher* 29 (2–3), 135–142.

DiNapoli, R. (2003) Towards natural engagement in non-exhibitional dramatic role-plays. *Iberica* 6, 15–38.

Dogra, N. and Wass, V. (2006) Can we assess students' awareness of cultural diversity? A qualitative study of stakeholders' views. *Medical Education* 40, 682–690.

Dolev, J.C., Friedlander, L.K. and Braverman, I. (2001) Use of fine art to enhance visual diagnostic skills. *Journal of the American Medical Association* 286 (9), 1020–1021.

Duffy, S. (2002) Intercultural competencies of upper secondary school learners of French. PhD thesis: University of Durham.

Eleftheriadou, Z., Lloyd, M. and Bor, R. (2009) Guidelines on communicating with children and young people. In M. Lloyd and R. Bor (eds) (2009) *Communication Skills for Medicine* (3rd edn) (pp. 111–126). London: Elsevier.

Eva, K.W. (2001) Assessing tutorial assessment. *Advances in Health Sciences Education* 6 (3), 243–257.

Evans, M. and Finlay, I. (eds) (2001) *Medical Humanities*. London: BMJ Books.

Evans, M., Ahlzén, R., Heath, I. and MacNaughton, J. (eds) (2008) *Medical Humanities Vol. 1: Symptom*. Abingdon: Radcliffe.

Fadiman, A. (1998) *The Spirit Catches You and You Fall Down*. New York: Farrar, Strauss and Giroux.

Fan, A., Chen, C., Su, T., Shih, W., Lee, C. and Hou, S. (2007) The association between parental socioeconomic status (SES) and medical students' personal and professional development. *Annals, Academy of Medicine, Singapore* 36 (9), 735–742.

Ferguson, G. (2001) If you pop over there: a corpus-based study of conditionals in medical discourse. *English for Specific Purposes* 20 (1), 61–82.

Fontanarosa, P.B. and Lundberg, G.D. (1998) Alternative medicine meets science. *Journal of the American Medical Association* 280 (18), 1618–1619.

Fotos, S. (1993) Consciousness-raising and noticing through focus on form: Grammar task performance vs. formal instruction. *Applied Linguistics* 14 (4), 385–407.

Fotos, S. and Ellis, R. (1991) Communicating about grammar: A task-based approach. *TESOL Quarterly* 25 (4), 605–628.

Foucault, M. (1979) *Discipline and Punish: The Birth of the Prison*, trans. A. Sheridan, London: Allen Lane.

Foucault, M. (1980) *Power/Knowledge: Selected Interviews and Other Writings, 1972–1977*, Colin Gordon (ed.). Harvester: London.

Freire, P. (1970) *Pedagogy of the Oppressed*, trans. M. Bergman. London: Penguin.

Friedman, L.D. (2002) The precarious position of the medical humanities in the medical school curriculum. *Academic Medicine 77*, 320–322.

Garfinkel, H. (1967) *Studies in Ethnomethodology*. Englewood Cliffs, NJ: Prentice-Hall.

Gavioli, L. (2002) Some thoughts on the problem of representing ESP through small corpora. In B. Ketteman and G. Marko (eds) *Language and Computers: Studies in Practical Linguistics* (pp. 293–303). Amsterdam: Rodopi.

General Medical Council [GMC] (1993, revised 2003, 2009) *Tomorrows Doctors: Recommendations on Undergraduate Medical Education* London: General Medical Council. [Retrieved from http://www.gmc-uk.org/TomorrowsDoctors_2003.pdf_39262074.pdf and http://www.gmc-uk.org/static/documents/content/TomorrowsDoctors_2009.pdf]

Genessee, F. (2001) Evaluation. In R. Carter and D. Nunan (eds) (2001) *The Cambridge Guide to Teaching English to Speakers of Other Languages* (pp. 144–150). Cambridge: Cambridge University Press.

Ghadessy, M. (ed.) (1988) *Registers of Written English: Situational Factors and Linguistic Features*. London: Pinter.

Giroux, H. (1992) *Border Crossings: Cultural Workers and the Politics of Education*. London: Routledge.

Giroux, H. (2001) *Theory and Resistance in Education*. Westport, CT: Bergin and Garvey.

Glasser, B. (2005) Magic bullets, dark victories and cold comforts: Some preliminary observations about stories of sickness in the cinema. In G. Harper and A. Moor (eds) *Signs of Life: Medicine and Cinema* (pp. 7–18). London: Wallflower Press.

Glendinning, E. and Holmström, B. (2005) *English in Medicine: A Course in Communications Skills* (3rd edn). Cambridge: Cambridge University Press.

Glendinning, E.H. and Howard, R. (2007) *Professional English in Use: Medicine*. Cambridge: Cambridge University Press.

Gokhale, A. (1995) Collaborative learning enhances critical thinking. *Journal of Technology Education 7* (1), 22–30.

Goldstein, B. (2009) *Working with Images: A Resource Book for the Language Classroom*. Cambridge: Cambridge University Press.

Gordon, J.J. and Evans, H.M. (2010) Learning medicine from the humanities. In T. Swanwick (ed.) *Understanding Medical Education: Evidence, Theory and Practice* (pp. 83–98). Oxford: Wiley-Blackwell.

Goulston, S.J.M. (2001). Medical education in 2001: The place of the Medical Humanities. *Internal Medicine Journal 31* (2), 123–127.

Griffiths, C. (ed.) (2008) *Lessons from Good Language Learners*. Cambridge: Cambridge University Press.

Guilherme, M. (2002) *Critical Citizens for an Intercultural World*. Clevedon: Multilingual Matters.

Guo, C. (1987) A needs study of undergraduate and graduate EST students and in-service technical professionals. *Papers from the fourth conference on English teaching and learning in the Republic of China* (pp. 263–274). Taipei: Crane.

Hafferty, F.W. (2006) Professionalism – the next wave. *The New England Journal of Medicine 356*, 2151–2152.

Hall, G. (2005) *Literature in Language Teaching*. London: Palgrave Macmillan.

Halkowski, T. (2011) Medical discourse. In K. Hyland and B. Paltridge (eds) *The Continuum Companion to Discourse Analysis* (pp. 321–332). London and New York: Continuum.

Halliday, M.A.K., McIntosh, A. and Strevens, P. (1964) *The Linguistic Sciences and Language Teaching*. London: Longman.

Halliday, M.A.K. and Hasan, R. (1985) *Text and Context: Aspects of Language in a Social-Semiotic Perspective*. Victoria: Deakin University Press.

Harper, G. and Moor, A. (eds) (2005) *Signs of Life: Medicine and Cinema*. London: Wallflower Press.

Harvard University (2007) *Report of the Task Force on General Education*. Faculty of Arts and Science, accessed 27 April 2012. http://www.sp07.umd.edu/HarvardGeneralEducation Report.pdf

Harvey, K.J., Brown, B., Crawford, P., Macfarlane, A. and McPherson, A. (2007) Am I normal? Teenagers, sexual health and the internet. *Social Science and Medicine* 65 (4), 771–781.

Hasselkus, B.R. (1992) The family caregiver as interpreter in the geriatric medical interview. *Medical Anthropology Quarterly*, New Series 6 (3), 288–304.

Hawkins, A.H. and McEntyre, M.C. (eds) (2000) *Teaching Literature and Medicine*. New York: Modern Languages Association of America.

Hayes, S.C. and Farnill, D. (1993) Medical training and English language proficiency. *Medical Education* 27 (1), 6–14.

Hemingway, E. (1966) *The Short Stories of Ernest Hemingway*. New York: Scribner's.

Heritage, J. and Stivers, T. (1999) Online commentary in acute medical visits: A method of shaping patient expectations. *Social Science and Medicine* 49, 1501–1517.

Ho, M-J. (2003) An example of medical humanities education. *Chung-Wai Literary Monthly* 31 (12), 11–25.

Hofstede, G. (2005) *Cultures and Organizations: Software of the Mind*. New York: McGraw-Hill.

Huang, C. (1980) *The Drowning of an Old Cat and Other Stories*, trans. H. Goldblatt, Bloomington: Indiana University Press.

Huang, C.J. (2002) The significance of General Education in the Reform of Medical Education: An Exploration of University General Education: Taiwan's Experience and its Implications. pp. 131–156.

Huang, Y. and Lin, S. (2010) A study of medical students' linguistic needs in Taiwan. *Asian ESP Journal* Spring, 35–58 [Retrieved from http://www.asian-esp-journal.com/ May_2010_Ebook.pdf].

Hunston, S. (2002) *Corpora in Applied Linguistics*. Cambridge: Cambridge University Press.

Hussain, R.M.R., Mamat, W.H.W., Salleh, N., Saat, R.M. and Harland, T. (2007) Problem-based learning in Asian Universities. *Studies in Higher Education* 32 (6), 761–772.

Hutchinson, T. and Waters, A. (1987) *English for Specific Purposes: A Learning-centred Approach*. Cambridge: Cambridge University Press.

Hyland, T. (1997) Reconsidering competence. *Journal of the Philosophy of Education Society of Great Britain* 31 (3), 491–503.

Hyland, K. (2000) *Disciplinary Discourses: Social Interactions in Academic Writing*. Harlow: Longman.

Hyland, K. (2002) Specificity revisited: how far should we go? *English for Specific Purposes* 21 (4), 385–395.

Hyland, K. (2006) *English for Academic Purposes: An Advanced Resource Book*. London: Routledge.

Hyland, K. and Paltridge, B. (eds) (2011) *The Continuum Companion to Discourse Analysis*. London and New York: Continuum.

Hyland, K. and Tse, P. (2007) Is there an "academic vocabulary"? *TESOL Quarterly* 41 (2), 235–254.

Hymes, D.H. (1971) *On Communicative Competence*. Philadelphia: University of Pennsylvania Press.

Ijpma, F.F.A. *et al.* (2006) The anatomy lesson of Dr. Nicolaes Tulp by Rembrandt (1632): A comparison of the painting with a dissected left forearm of a dutch male cadaver. *Journal of Hand Surgery* 31 (6), 882–891.

Jobson, M.R. and Knapp van Bogaert, D. (2005) Just a story or a 'just' story? Ethical issues in a film with a medical theme. In G. Harper and A. Moor (eds) (2005) *Signs of Life: Medicine and Cinema* (pp. 82–91). London: Wallflower Press.

Jones, A. (2003) Nurses talking to patients: exploring conversation analysis as a means of researching nurse-patient communication. *International Journal of Nursing Studies* 40, 609–618.

Jones, A. (2009) Creating history: documents and patient participation in nurse-patient interviews. *Sociology of Health and Illness* 31 (6), 907–923.

Kachur, E.K. and Altshuler, L. (2004) Cultural competence is everyone's responsibility! *Medical Teacher* 26 (2), 101–105.

Kleinman, A. (1980) *Patients and Healers in the Context of Culture*. Berkeley: University of California Press.

Kleinman, A. (1988) *The Illness Narratives: Suffering, Healing, and the Human Condition*. New York: Basic Books.

Krane, D. (2005) Number of 'cyberchondriacs' – US adults who go online for health information – increases to estimated 117. *Healthcare News* 8 (5). [Retrieved from http://www.harrisinteractive.com/news/newsletters_healthcare.asp] 27th April 2012.

Kripalani, S., Bussey-Jones, J., Katz, M. G. and Genao, I. (2006) A prescription for cultural competence in medical education. *Journal of General Internal Medicine* 21 (1), 116–1120.

Khoo, H.E. (2003) Implementation of problem-based learning in Asian medical schools and students perceptions of their experience. *Medical Education* 37 (5), 401–409.

Kohler, J. (1991) Interviewing and counselling children and their families. In R. Corney (ed.) *Developing Communication and Counselling Skills in Medicine* (pp. 87–96). London and New York: Tavistock/Routledge.

Kramsch, C. (1993) *Context and Culture in Language Teaching*. Oxford: Oxford University Press.

Kress, G. and van Leeuwen, T. (1996) *Reading Images: The Grammar of visual Design*. London: Routledge.

Kubetin, S.K. (2002) Yale students now study art as well as medicine. *Skin and Allergy News*. June issue. [Retrieved from http://findarticles.com/p/articles/mi_hb4393/is_6_33/ai_n28925711]

Kumaravadivelu, B. (1993) The name of the task and the task of naming: Methodological aspects of task-based pedagogy. In G. Crookes and S. Gass (eds) *Tasks in a Pedagogical Context* (pp. 69–96). Clevedon: Multilingual Matters.

Kumaravadivelu, B. (2006) TESOL methods: Changing tracks, challenging trends. *TESOL Quarterly* 40 (1), 59–81.

Kumaş-Tan, Z., Beagan, B., Loppie, C., MacLeod, A. and Blye, F. (2007) Measures of cultural competence: Examining hidden assumptions. *Academic Medicine* 82 (6), 548–557.

Kushner, T. ([1992, 1993] 2007) *Angels in America: A Gay Fantasia on National Themes. Part One: Millennium Approaches; Part Two: Perestroika*. London: Nick Hern Books.

Kwong, T.Y., Kwong, Q., O'Brien, A., Haswell, J. and Hill, K. (2009) *Medical Communication Skills and Law: The Patient Centred Approach Made Easy*. Edinburgh: Churchill Livingstone Elsevier.

Lahtinen, A-M. and Torppa, M. (2007) "Medicalisation of falling in love": medical students' reponses to Thomas Mann's The Black Swan. *Journal of Medical Ethics; Medical Humanities* 33, 44–48.

Lai, J. (1997) *Reading Strategies: A Study Guide*. Hong Kong: Chinese University of Hong Kong.

Landsborough, M. (1932) *More Stories from Formosa*. London: Presbyterian Church of England, Publications Committee.

Landsborough, M. (1957) *Dr. Lan: A Short Biography of Dr. David Landsborough, Medical Missionary of the Presbyterian Church of England in Formosa, 1895-1936*. London: Presbyterian Church of England, Publications Committee.

Lazar, G. (1993) *Literature and Language Teaching: A Guide for Teachers and Trainers*. Cambridge: Cambridge University Press.

Lázár, I., Huber-Kriegler, M., Lussier, D., Matei, G.S. and Peck, C. (eds) (2007) *Developing and Assessing Intercultural Communicative Competence: A Guide for Language Teachers and Teacher Educators*. Strasbourg: Council of Europe.

Lazarus, E. (1988) Theoretical considerations for the study of the doctor-patient relationship: implications of a perinatal study. *Medical Anthropology Quarterly* 2 (1), 34–58.

Lee, R.K.M.W. and Kwan, C. (1997) The use of problem-based learning in medical education. *Journal of Medical Education* 1 (2), 149–157.

Levine, G.S. and Phipps, A. (eds) (2010) *Critical and Intercultural Theory and Language Pedagogy*. American Association of University Supervisors, Coordinators and Directors of Foreign Language Programs [AAUSC] Issues in Language Program Direction, 2010, Boston: Heinle.

Li Wei (1994) *Three Generations Two Languages One Family: Language Choice and Language Shift in a Chinese Community in Britain*. Clevedon: Multilingual Matters.

Li Wei (2002) 'What do you want me to say?' On the conversation analysis approach to bilingual interaction. *Language in Society* 31 (2), 159–180.

Lie, D.A, Boker, J. and Cleveland, E. (2006) Using the *Tool for Assessing Cultural Competence Training* (TACCT) to measure faculty and medical student perceptions of cultural competence instruction in the first three years of the curriculum. *Academic Medicine* 81 (6), 557–564.

Lieberman, P. (1963) Some effects of semantic and grammatical context on the production and perception of speech. *Language and Speech* 6, 172–187.

Little, D. (2002) The European Language Portfolio: structure, origins, implementation and challenges. *Language Teaching* 35 (3), 182–189.

Lloyd, M. and Bor, R. (2009) *Communication Skills for Medicine* (3rd edn). London: Elsevier.

Lock, M. (1980) *East Asian Medicine in Urban Japan: Varieties of Medical Experience*. Berkeley: University of California Press.

Long, M.H. (ed.) (2005) *Second Language Needs Analysis*. Cambridge: Cambridge University Press.

Long, M.H. and Crookes, G. (1992) Three approaches to task-based language teaching. *TESOL Quarterly* 26 (1), 27–56.

Lu, P. (2006) Developing an Intercultural English Curriculum at University Level in Taiwan. Unpublished PhD thesis: University of Glasgow.

Lu, P. (2010) Medicine as art: An interview with Christine Borland. *Language and Intercultural Communication* 10 (1), 90–99.

Lu, P. and Corbett, J. (2010) The health care professional as intercultural speaker. In G.S. Levine and A. Phipps (eds) *Critical and Intercultural Theory and Language Pedagogy*. American Association of University Supervisors, Coordinators and Directors of Foreign Language Programs [AAUSC] Issues in Language Program Direction, 2010, Boston: Heinlepp. pp. 76–94.

Lucas, P., Lenstrup, M., Prinz, J., Williamson, D., Yip, H. and Tipoe, G. (1997) Language as a barrier to the acquisition of anatomical knowledge. *Medical Education* 31 (2), 81–86.

Lupton, D. (2003) *Medicine as Culture* (2nd edn). London: Sage.

MacRae, J. (1991) *Literature with a Small 'l'*. London: Macmillan.

McEntyre, M.C. (2000) Touchstones: A brief survey of some standard works. In A.H. Hawkins and M.C. McEntyre (eds) *Teaching Literature and Medicine* (pp. 187–199). New York: Modern Languages Association of America.

McNeill, W.H. (1976) *Plagues and Peoples*. New York: Doubleday.

Maher, J. (1986) The development of English as an international language of medicine. *Applied Linguistics* 7 (2), 206–218.

Mangione-Smith, R., Stivers, T., Elliott, M., McDonald, L. and Heritage, J. (2003) Online commentary during the physical examination: a communication tool for avoiding inappropriate antibiotic prescribing? *Social Science and Medicine* 56, 313–320.

Marshall, R. and Bleakley, A. (2009) The death of Hector: Pity in Homer, empathy in medical education. *Medical Humanities* 35 (1), 7–12.

Martin, E. (1991) The egg and the sperm: How science has constructed a romance based on stereotypical male-female roles. *Signs: Journal of Women in Culture and Society* 16 (3), 485–501.

Members of the Medical Professionalism Project (2002) Medical Professionalism in the new millennium: A physician charter. *Annals of Internal Medicine* 136 (3), 243–246.

Met, M. and Byram, M. (1999) Standards for foreign language learning and the teaching of culture. *Language Learning Journal* 19, 61–68.

Montgomery, M., Durant, A., Fabb, N., Furniss, T. and Mills, S. (2007) *Ways of Reading: Advanced Reading Skills for Students of English Literature* (3rd edn). London: Routledge.

Moss, B. and Roberts, C. (2003) *Doing the Lambeth Talk: Real-Life GP-Patient Encounters in the Multi-Lingual City* (DVD and booklet). London: Kings College/London Deanery.

Moss, B. and Roberts, C. (2005) Explanations, explanations, explanations: How do patients with limited English construct narrative accounts in multi-lingual, multi-ethnic settings and how can GPs interpret them? *Family Practice* 22, 412–418.

Mpofu, D.J.S., Lanphear, J., Stewart, T., Das, M., Ridding, P. and Dunn, E. (1998) Facility with the English language and problem-based learning group interaction: Findings from an Arabic setting. *Medical Education* 32 (5), 479–485.

Munby, J. (1978) *Communicative Syllabus Design*. Cambridge: Cambridge University Press.

National Standards in Foreign Language Education Project (1999, 2006) *Standards for Foreign Language Learning in the 21st Century*, (2nd and 3rd edns). Lawrence, KS: Allen Press.

Neuner, G. and Byram, M. (eds) (2003) *Intercultural Competence* Vol. 1, Strasbourg: Council of Europe.

Nunan, D. (1989) *Designing Tasks for the Communicative Classroom*. Cambridge: Cambridge University Press.

Nunan, D. (2004) *Task-based Language Teaching*. Cambridge: Cambridge University Press. [A revised edition of Nunan, 1989].

Nation, I.S.P. and Macalister, J. (2010) *Language Curriculum Design*. London: Routledge.

Nwogu, K.N. (1991) Structure of science popularizations: A genre-analysis approach to the schema of popularized medical texts. *English for Specific Purposes* 10 (2), 111–123.

Nwogu, K.N. (1997) The medical research paper: Structure and functions. *English for Specific Purposes* 16 (2), 119–138.

Nwogu, K.N. and Bloor, T. (1991) Thematic progression in professional and popular medical texts. In E. Ventola (ed.) *Functional and Systemic Linguistics: Approaches and Uses* (pp. 369–384). Berlin and New York: Mouton de Gruyter.

O'Dowd, R. (ed.) (2007) *Online Intercultural Exchange: An Introduction for Foreign Language Teachers*. Clevedon: Multilingual Matters.

O'Keeffe, A., McCarthy, M. and Carter, R. (2007) *From Corpus to Classroom: Language Use and Language Teaching*. Cambridge: Cambridge University Press.

Phipps, A. and Levine, G.S. (2010) What is language pedagogy for? In G.S. Levine and A. Phipps (eds) *Critical and Intercultural Theory and Language Pedagogy* (pp. 1–14). American Association of University Supervisors, Coordinators and Directors of Foreign Language Programs [AAUSC] Issues in Language Program Direction, 2010, Boston: Heinle.

Pomerance, B. (1979) *The Elephant Man*. New York: Grove Press.

Porter, R. (1999) *The Greatest Benefit to Mankind: A Medical History of Humanity from Antiquity to the Present*. New York: WW Norton.

Porter, R. (2005) *Flesh in the Age of Reason*. New Edition, London: Penguin.

Posner, T. (1991) What's in a smear? Cervical screening, medical signs and metaphors. *Science as Culture* 2 (2), 160–187.

Potter, J. (1996) *Representing Reality. Discourse, Rhetoric and Social Construction*. London: Sage.

Prabhu, N.S. (1987) *Second Language Pedagogy*. Oxford: Oxford University Press.

Prewitt, K.W. (2000) Teaching the body in texts: Literature, culture and religion. In A.H. Hawkins and M.C. McEntyre (eds) *Teaching Literature and Medicine* (pp. 77–91). New York: Modern Languages Association of America.

Rapp, D.E. (2006) Integrating cultural competency into the undergraduate medical curriculum. *Medical Education* 40 (7), 704–710.

Rees, C. and Ruiz, S. (2003) *Compendium of Cultural Competence Initiatives in Healthcare*. Washington, DC: The Henry J. Kaiser Family Foundation.

Reynolds, R. and Stone, J. (eds) (1995) *On Doctoring: Poems, Stories, Essays*. Revised edn. New York: Simon and Schuster.

Richards, J.C. and Rodgers, T.S. (2001) *Approaches and Methods in Language Teaching*. Cambridge: Cambridge University Press.

Ridgway, T. (2000) Listening strategies – I beg your pardon? *ELT Journal* 54 (2), 179–185.

Risager, K. (2007) *Language and Culture Pedagogy*. Clevedon: Multilingual Matters.

Roberts, C. (1997) Transcribing talk: Issues of representation. *TESOL Quarterly* 31 (1), 167–172.

Roberts, C., Atwell, C., Swanwick, T. and Chana, N. (2008) *Words in Action: Communication Skills for Doctors New to UK General Practice* (DVD and booklet). London: Kings College/London Deanery.

Roberts, C., Byram, M., Barro, A., Jordan, S. and Street, B. (2001) *Language Learners as Ethnographers*. Clevedon: Multilingual Matters.

Roberts, C., Sarangi, S., Southgate, L., Wakeford, R. and Wass, V. (2000) Oral examinations—equal opportunities, ethnicity, and fairness in the MRCGP. *BMJ* 320 (5 February), 370–375.

Roberts, J., Sanders, T. and Wass, V. (2008) Students' perceptions of race, ethnicity and culture at two UK medical schools. *Medical Education* 42 (1), 45–52.

Rosow, I. (1981) Coalitions in geriatric medicine. In M.R. Haug (ed.) *Elderly Patients and Their Doctors* (pp. 137–146). New York: Springer.

Rutherford, W.E. (1987) *Second Language Grammar: Learning and Teaching*. London and New York: Longman.

Salinsky, J. (2002) *Medicine and Literature: The Doctor's Companion to the Classics*. Vol. 1. Abingdon: Radcliffe.

Sarangi, S. and Roberts, C. (1999) *Talk, Work and Institutional Order: Discourse in Medical, Mediation and Management Settings*. Berlin: Mouton de Gruyter.

Seeleman, C., Suurmond, J. and Stronks, K. (2009) Cultural competence: A conceptual framework for teaching and learning. *Medical Education* 43 (3), 229–237.

Shapiro, J. (2006) A sampling of the medical humanities. *Journal for Learning through the Arts* 2 (1). [Retrieved from http://escholarship.org/uc/item/58b5h3h9]

Shapiro, J., Coulehan, J., Wear, D. and Montello, M. (2009) Medical humanities and their discontents: Definitions, critiques, and implications. *Academic Medicine* 84 (2), 192–198.

Shem, S. (1978) *The House of God*. New York: Bantam Doubleday.

Shi, L. (2009) English for medical purposes. In D. Belcher (ed.) (2009) *English for Specific Purposes in Theory and Practice* (pp. 205–228). Ann Arbor: University of Michigan Press.

Shi, L, Corcos, R. and Storey, A. (2001) Using student performance data to develop an English course for clinical training. *English for Specific Purposes* 20, 267–291.

Shields, H. (2008) Integrating cross cultural care into a pre-clinical science course: A faculty development program for tutors. Presentation given at a conference on *Cultural Competence in Medical Education*, Kaohsiung Medical University, November 15 2008.

Sim, S.M., Azila, N.M., Lian, L.H., Tan, C.P. and Tan, N.H. (2006) A simple instrument for the assessment of student performance in problem-based learning tutorials. *Annals of the Academy of Medicine, Singapore* 35 (9), 634–641. [Retrieved from http://www.annals.edu.sg/pdf/35VolNo9Sep2006/V35N9p634.pdf].

Simmel, G. (1950) *The Sociology of Georg Simmel*, trans. K.H. Wolf. New York: Free Press.

Skelton, J. (2008) *Language and Clinical Communication: This Bright Babylon*. Oxford and New York: Radcliffe.

Skelton, J., Murray, J. and Hobbs, F.D.R. (1999) Imprecision in medical communication: Study of a doctor talking to patients with serious illness. *Journal of the Royal Society of Medicine* 92, 620–625.

Skelton, J., Thomas, C.P. and Macleod, J.A.A. (2000a) Teaching literature and medicine to medical students, part I: The beginning. *Lancet* 356 (Dec 2), 1920–1922.

Skelton, J., Thomas, C.P. and Macleod, J.A.A. (2000b) Teaching literature and medicine to medical students, part I: The beginning. *Lancet* 356 (Dec 9), 2001–2003.

Solzhenitsyn, A. (1968) *Cancer Ward* (Alexander Dolberg trans.). London: Bodley Head.

Sontag, S. (2002) *Illness as Metaphor and AIDS and its Metaphors*. New York: Picador. [A republication of *Illness as Metaphor* (1978) and *AIDS and its Metaphors* (1989).]

Stein, H. (1990) *American Medicine as Culture*. Boulder, CO: Westview.

Stern, D.T. and Papadakis, M. (2006) The developing physician – becoming a professional. *The New England Journal of Medicine* 355, 1794–1799.

Stjernquist, M. and Crang-Svalenius, E. (2007) Applying the case method for teaching within the health professions – teaching the students. *Education for Health* 15 http://www.educationforhealth.net (accessed 28 September 2009).

Stoner, B.P. (1986) Understanding medical systems: Traditional, modern, and syncretic health care alternatives in medically pluralistic societies. *Medical Anthropology Quarterly* 17 (2), 44–48.

Strathern, A. and Stewart, P.J. (1999) *Curing and Healing: Medical Anthropology in Global Perspective*. Durham: Carolina University Press.

Surawicz, B. and Jacobson, B. (eds) (2009) *Doctors in Fiction: Lessons from Literature*. Abingdon: Radcliffe.

Svendsen, C. and Krebs, K. (1984) Identifying English for the job: Examples from health care occupations. *English for Specific Purposes* 3, 153–164.

Swales, J. (1990) *Genre Analysis: English in Academic and Research Settings*. Cambridge: Cambridge University Press.

Swanwick, T. (ed.) (2010) *Understanding Medical Education: Evidence, Theory and Practice*. Oxford: Wiley-Blackwell.

Taavitsainen, I. and Pahta, P. (eds) (2011) *Medical Writing in Early Modern English*. Cambridge: Cambridge University Press.

Teal, C.R. and Street, R.L. (2009) Critical elements of culturally competent communication in the medical encounter: A review and model. *Social Science and Medicine* 68, 533–543.

Tervalon, M. and Murray-García, J. (1998) Cultural humility versus cultural competence: A critical distinction in defining physician training outcomes in multicultural education. *Journal of Health Care for the Poor and Underserved* 9 (2), 117–125.

Tessmer, M. (1990) Environment analysis: A neglected stage of instructional design. *Educational Technology Research and Development* 38 (1), 55–64.

Thiong'o, N.W. (1986) *Decolonising the Mind: The Politics of Language in African Literature*. Nairobi: East African Educational Publishers.

Thornborrow, J. and Wareing, S. (1998) *Patterns in Language: An Introduction to Language and Literary Style*. London: Routledge.

Thurlow, C., Tomic, A. and Lengel, L.B. (2004) *Computer Mediated Communication: Social Interaction and the Internet*. Thousand Oaks, CA: Sage.

Trompenaars, F. and Hampden-Turner, C. (1998) *Riding the Waves of Culture: Understanding Cultural Diversity in Business* (2nd edn). New York: McGraw-Hill.

Turner, B. (1996) *The Body and Society: Explorations in Social Theory*. 2nd edn. London: Sage.

University of Washington Medical Center (2007) Communicating with your Chinese patient. [Retrieved from http://depts.washington.edu/pfes/PDFs/ChineseCultureClue.pdf]

Valle, R., Petra, L., Martínez-Gonzáez, A., Rojas-Ramirez, J.A., Morales-Lopez, S. and Piña-Garza, B. (1999) Assessment of student performance in problem-based learning tutorial sessions. *Medical Education* 33 (11), 818–822.

Van den Branden, K. (ed.) (2006) *Task-Based Language Education*. Cambridge: Cambridge University Press.

Vosnesenskaya, J. (1986) *The Women's Decameron*, trans. W.B. Linton. New York: Henry Holt.

Wald, P. (2008) *Contagious: Cultures, Carriers and the Outbreak Narrative*. Durham NC and London: Duke University Press.

Wall, D. (2010) Evaluation: Improving practice, influencing policy. In T. Swanwick (ed.) (2010) *Understanding Medical Education: Evidence, Theory and Practice* (pp. 336–351). Oxford: Wiley-Blackwell.

Warschauer, M. and Kern, R. (eds) (2000) *Network-based Language Teaching: Concepts and practice*. Cambridge: Cambridge University Press.

Wass, V., Roberts, C., Hoogenboom, R., Jones, R. and Van der Vleuten, C. (2003) Effect of ethnicity on performance in a final objective structured clinical examination: Qualitative and quantitative study. *British Medical Journal* 326, 800–803.

Watson, R., Stimpson, A., Topping, A. and Porock, D. (2002) Clinical competence assessment in nursing: As systematic review of the literature. *Journal of Advanced Nursing* 39 (5), 421–431.

Wenger, E. (1998) *Communities of Practice: Learning, Meaning and Identity.* Cambridge: Cambridge University Press.

West, R. (1994) Needs analysis in language teaching. *Language Teaching* 27 (1), 1–19.

Weston, G (2009) *Direct Red: A Surgeons Story.* London: Jonathan Cape.

Williams, I. (1996) A contextual study of lexical verbs in two types of medical research report: Clinical and Experimental. *English for Specific Purposes* 15 (3), 175–197.

Willis, D. and Willis, J. (2001) Task-based language learning. In R. Carter and D. Nunan (eds) *The Cambridge Guide to Teaching English to Speakers of Other Languages* (pp. 173–178). Cambridge: Cambridge University Press.

Worsley, P. (1982) Non-Western medical systems. *Annual Review of Anthropology* 11, 315–348.

Wright, A. (1990) *Pictures for Language Learning.* Cambridge: Cambridge University Press.

Wu, H.Y-J. (2008) Between God's Miracle and Imperialist's Propaganda: Love of a Skin-graft (1928) Revisited. Paper presented at the Fifth Conference of the European Association of Taiwan Studies, Charles University, Prague: 18–20 April. [Retrieved from http://www.soas.ac.uk/taiwanstudies/eats/eats2008/file43184.pdf]

# Index

*Note:* 'n' denotes note

For Product Safety Concerns and Information please contact our EU Authorised Representative:

Easy Access System Europe

Mustamäe tee 50

10621 Tallinn

Estonia

gpsr.requests@easproject.com